Antenatal Education

Antenatal Education
GUIDELINES FOR TEACHERS

Margaret Williams MCSP MAOT,
Obstetric Physiotherapist,
Advanced Teacher of the National Childbirth Trust

Dorothy Booth SRN SCM HV FWT
Health Visitor and Fieldwork Teacher,
Richmond, Twickenham and Roehampton Health Authority, Surrey.
Advanced Teacher of the National Childbirth Trust

FOREWORD BY

Professor Philip Rhodes
MA MB FRCS FRCOG
Professor of Postgraduate Medical Education,
University of Southampton, and Dean of
Graduate Medicine for the Wessex Region

THIRD EDITION

CHURCHILL LIVINGSTONE
EDINBURGH LONDON MELBOURNE AND NEW YORK 1985

CHURCHILL LIVINGSTONE
Medical Division of Longman Group Limited

Distributed in the United States of America by
Churchill Livingstone Inc., 1560 Broadway, New York,
N.Y. 10036, and by associated companies, branches and
representatives throughout the world.

First Edition 1974
Second Edition 1980
Third Edition 1985

ISBN 0 443 03015 4

British Library Cataloguing in Publication Data
Williams, Margaret, *1915*–
 Antenatal education.—3rd ed.
 1. Childbirth—Study and teaching
 I. Title II. Booth, Dorothy
 618.2'4 RG973

Library of Congress Cataloging in Publication Data
Williams, Margaret, *1915*–
 Antenatal education.
 Includes bibliographical references and index.
 1. Childbirth—Study and teaching. I. Booth,
Dorothy, S.R.N. II. Title.
RG973.W54 1984 618.2'4'071 83–15028

Printed in Singapore by The Print House (Pte) Ltd

Foreword

Falling maternal mortality and perinatal mortality rates demonstrate improvements in the prognosis for childbearing. Obstetric and midwifery practice has helped with this improvement, though there are other factors such as housing, education and nutrition, as well as sanitation which may have made at least as large an impact on the physical results. As standards of care rise in obstetrics, it is right and natural that mothers expect more of the maternity services. One aspect of this increased expectancy is seen in the demand for 'natural childbirth', 'relaxation classes', 'psychoprophylaxis', 'preparation for childbirth'; it scarcely matters what it is called. Mothers want psychological help and support through pregnancy, labour and afterwards. They want to know what is going on. And they have a right to know for they are actively involved and not passive ciphers. Those who look after and care for childbearing women know how valuable it is for these mothers to be intelligently aware of their bodies and physiological processes, and for them to learn of relationships with their babies and husbands and other members of their families. In the present climate of opinion it is no longer necessary to defend antenatal education.

There is a problem, however, in arranging for education. It is time-consuming, needs small group teaching and continuous boundless enthusiasm from the teachers. In England and Wales there are over 700 000 births each year. Providing good education antenatally for all these mothers is a herculean task which requires a large work force. And this is no field for the enthusiastic amateur teacher, full of myths and prejudices, and with unswerving allegiance to harebrained theories, hypotheses and 'systems'. The antenatal educator must be a professional with a balanced outlook and a deep knowledge of pregnancy, labour, babies and, above all, of human psychology and individual variability, and she must have qualities of perceptiveness, tact and sympathy.

The prescription for a good antenatal teacher is compounded of human qualities, knowledge and skills, the last being needed to project the message of helpful education. Education is not didactic teaching. It is tailoring what is taught to the needs of the individual mother so that she may understand within her own intellectual capacity.

There have been many books and pamphlets on antenatal preparation, but none, until this one, which will teach the teachers. It is balanced and thoughtful and is based upon the extensive practical experience of both the authors. It is especially valuable for its survey of teaching methods and aims, and no antenatal educator can afford to ignore the wise advice given here on how to get information across to a disparate group, and on how to draw out such a group so that its fears, tensions, emotions and anxieties can be verbalised.

As befits two such excellent educators the books is without dogma. It suggests and hints and subtly makes the reader *think* about the whole of antenatal education, whilst at the same time it offers really practical advice. I would like it to be read and understood by all with pretensions to antenatal teaching, for then its enlightened and humane philosophy will be disseminated to thousands of women who will benefit.

P.R.

Preface to the Third Edition

Further developments, improved technological management such as better methods of monitoring the fetus, improved analgesia and shortening of labour have naturally occurred. On the other hand, new evidence has proved that making use of the mother's natural resources, a more humane attitude to the management of labour and less intervention leads to more comfortable and shorter labours. If teachers believe this evidence and wish to teach mothers to trust in their own instincts it is not always easy for them to prepare women for more conventional management without disloyalty to colleagues and the possibility of arousing conflicts between staff and parents at the vital time of labour.

In this edition we have tried to describe some of the new teaching and how it can be used, as well as how a teacher can help her group of parents to make the best use of more traditional care.

M.W.
D.B.

London, 1985

Preface to the First Edition

The perfect antenatal teacher would be a midwife, a health visitor, a physiotherapist, a psychologist and the mother of six children all born in different ways in different places. She would be something of an actress, a great enthusiast, have a deep interest in young people and a sense of humour. Such paragons do not exist, teachers are ordinary people who try to make the best use of their professional expertise and their life experiences. They listen to and learn from their students, the parents, and supplement their knowledge by discussion with colleagues and wide reading.

Teachers discover early in their first series of classes that it is one thing to acquire knowledge for an examination, quite another to pass on that knowledge to a group of people who have different backgrounds and need the information for a different purpose. They must be sure of their facts but able to differentiate clearly between facts and their own personal beliefs. This book has been written for those who have the required knowledge in one or other aspect of the work, in an attempt to guide them in the use of it in helping parents to understand childbirth and their reactions to it and to encourage them to make up their own minds what is best for their baby and themselves.

Some new teachers may have a mainly clinical background, in which case they need to observe and read more about the hopes, thoughts and fears of pregnant women, others, having recent personal experience of childbirth, may need to return to a more objective and professional outlook. Since at present there is no one full training which covers all aspects of antenatal education it is hoped that teachers will read about the aspects with which they are less familiar and may, perhaps, feel more competent to stand in, in the absence of a colleague.

Everyday language has been used throughout the book; more technical information will be found in other books listed in the bibliography. As methods of teaching depend so much on the personality of the teacher and a recapitulation of our full teaching programme would have been both lengthy and tedious, only guidelines and some check lists have been included. However, certain subjects which some teachers find difficult to put into words have been treated more fully. These passages of direct speech are shown in closely-set lines of type and may be useful until the teacher learns by trial and error to phrase them in her own language.

The information about books, equipment and audiovisual aids was correct at the time of going to press, but, as prices fluctuate, will need to be checked by each teacher.

Teaching and group leadership are vital skills, we have therefore chosen to describe the educators as teachers or leaders rather than by their qualifications.

London, 1974

M.W.
D.B.

Acknowledgements

We wish to thank Dr Andrew Gerard Doughty MB BS FFA RCS for his advice about epidural analgesia, and Miss Laura Mitchell MCSP DipL TP and Mrs Sheila Harrison MCSP for their contributions on their methods of teaching relaxation.

We gratefully acknowledge the contributions from overseas whose authors we have named. These contain resource lists from America, Australia, Canada and South Africa.

We are especially grateful to Professor Philip Rhodes MA MB FRCS FRCOG, Professor of Postgraduate Medical Education, University of Southampton, and Dean of Graduate Medicine for the Wessex Region, and Miss Judith Duffield SRN SCM MTD, Senior Nursing Officer (Teaching) Midwifery Division, Kingston Hospital, for reading the manuscript and for their helpful advice and criticism; to Mrs J Schiller BSc(Hons) SRD, Senior Dietitian, Barnet General Hospital for her advice on nutrition.

We also express our gratitude to our friends and colleagues, who have shared their ideas with us over the years, and especially to our antenatal class members, from whom we continue to learn.

If inadvertently we have used any teaching examples from sources we have not acknowledged we apologise for the omission.

Lastly, we thank our husbands and families for their forebearance and encouragement.

Contents

1 The aims and history of antenatal education   1
2 Teaching techniques   21
3 Audiovisual aids   43
4 Equipment and planning of classes   57
5 Discussion of pregnancy   71
6 Discussion of normal labour   104
7 Variations of labour patterns   147
8 Some new ideas   167
9 The puerperium and baby care   179
10 Fathers' evenings and film shows   207
11 The value of antenatal education   222

Appendix
Films, filmstrips, slides and useful addresses in the United Kingdom and overseas   234

Index   295

1

The aims and history of antenatal education

Men's and women's knowledge about childbirth and their attitudes towards birth and parenthood are conditioned by many factors. First, they are conditioned by their own parents, whether they have been loved and supported by them, yet freed as they grew up to develop along their own lines. Their attitudes are affected by how they have been disciplined, what they have observed and been taught about handling the situations arising in family life. Daughters may have learned that pregnancy is a normal consequence of marriage, the birth of a child a joyous achievement and the caring for that child a valued contribution to society. Equally, they may have learned that pregnancy is something that happens when you 'go wrong' or 'don't take care', birth is a painful and degrading experience and parenthood is of negligible value compared with other activities. Sons may have absorbed the message that bearing and rearing children is women's work and that men have more important things to do. These attitudes are further modified by other members of the cultural group who produce and talk about babies.

The next factor is more formal education, whether this comes from school, books, magazines or broadcasts. There has been a tremendous change in the last few years in the frequency with which birth is discussed and illustrated by the mass media, but this is coming more slowly in the schools. Nuffield science courses are improving the situation, but school biology still too frequently stops short at the rabbit or, at best, slides rapidly over human reproduction; it is rare to find a course which includes the emotional aspects and sensations of childbirth. In some schools parentcraft classes may offer valuable advice on bathing and caring for a baby but neglect opportunities for wider discussion on the responsibilities of parenthood, particularly in boys' schools. Recently the situation has improved and Perkins (1979) describes a school in the East Midlands where girls *and* boys spend half a day each week in a local nursery, a playgroup or at the mothers and toddlers club held in the school.

They are briefed on what to observe and discuss their findings with the teachers afterwards.

Finally, there is the personal interaction of the man and woman who conceive the child, perhaps as a planned and eagerly awaited fulfilment of their love, but perhaps as an unplanned 'mistake' which may offer a threat to an already unstable relationship.

AIMS

Teachers can observe and listen to these parents, trying to understand their differing attitudes and perhaps help them to understand how they have arisen. They can try to reinforce what they believe to be valuable and positive attitudes and to modify those that are less desirable. It is unlikely, however, in the few short weeks of an antenatal course that they will completely change beliefs that have taken 20 years to establish.

On being told that she is going to have a baby, a woman may be thrilled, distressed, confident or frightened or a mixture of all four. She rarely tries to analyse her feelings or to wonder how they have arisen. She is usually content to seek medical care and to make plans. She may be offered a course of preparation; what then do those who accept the offer hope to get out of the classes?

Most women, when asked, gave 'the desire to learn more about labour' as their primary reason for attending classes. We have had this view confirmed by informally questioning hundreds of mothers. The fathers want to know when they should take their wives to hospital or send for the midwife, and what they should do if the baby is born suddenly when the couple are alone. If one enquires a little more deeply what the women want to know they will often say 'it's not only the process of labour but how it will affect me, what "they" will do to me and how I can help myself and how I will be helped'. Similarly if the father intends to be present, he also wants to know what to expect of his wife and her attendants and particularly how he can help them.

Once assured that labour will be fully dealt with in the course, then women will ask for more information about pregnancy and the puerperium and more particularly about their babies. They seek help in understanding their bodily changes and emotional swings, in keeping as well and happy as possible during pregnancy, and in achieving full rehabilitation and fulfilment afterwards. Some want to know more of the development of their babies *in utero*, others prefer their own picture of events. Discussions on feeding and living habits planned to give the baby a good start in life, his appearance, and his needs for love, food and warmth are very popular subjects for discussion. The whole group likes to meet a young baby and exchange ideas with its mother.

Multigravid women come to classes either in the hope of achieving a better experience with another birth or because, having found a preparation course helpful during a first pregnancy, they wish for a refresher course. Some also seek help in planning their daily activities with a growing family and more particularly with helping another child to accept the new baby. They find it therapeutic to be able to relive their early days with their first babies thus helping primigravidae in the group to imagine their coming excitements, tiredness and ambivalence, and by sharing their experiences of this challenging period the multigravidae realise that they have changed and matured, and that for them their 'apprenticeship' is over.

During a first pregnancy a woman has to face tremendous changes in her life style. She will probably, at least temporarily, give up work, with its earnings, companionship and satisfactions and be restricted to her home environment where she may have no friends in the immediate neighbourhood. She and her partner will soon no longer be carefree young lovers responsible largely for themselves alone. The woman at least faces a seemingly complete loss of freedom and both are about to undertake the responsibility for the health and happiness of another human being, who appears fragile, utterly dependent and infinitely demanding. These parents often express a need to meet others undergoing similar experiences and wish to become part of this new peer group. They want to talk about their feelings and plans to one another and to a group leader who has preferably herself had the experience of childbirth and has both the time and a true wish to listen to them.

Summary of aims

These, as we see them, are:

1. The gradual building up of confidence in each woman in herself and in those who are looking after her; confidence acquired through knowledge, an understanding of her own reactions, and the ability to trust and control her own body.

2. To help her to have a healthy, happy pregnancy: healthy not only for the sake of the child but also so that there is a good basis for speedy physical rehabilitation postnatally; happy in looking

forward with joyful anticipation (even if with a little apprehension) to the birth.

3. That in labour she feels physically and mentally prepared for the reality that she meets and achieves a satisfying experience within the context of safe maternity care.

4. To provide a group whose members can air their thoughts and problems and work towards adjustment in their life styles.

5. To assist the bonding of the baby with its parents during the antenatal and immediate post partum phases; to begin to prepare for the physical and emotional care of that baby and to help the parents to accept it into their family setting. It is hoped that fathers will share in the preparation either indirectly through their wives' influence or directly by attending those parts of the course which are open to them, best of all by sharing the whole preparation at a couples' course.

6. Introducing the baby as a member of the family circle.

The teachers to achieve these aims

In hospital, even if the antenatal teaching is shared by midwives, physiotherapists, doctors and others, the achievement of common aims should only be a question of communication and mutual respect; teachers working in local authority and private classes have a more difficult task when trying to fulfil their roles as part of the team. Efforts to instil self-confidence in the parents must never be made at the expense of confidence in those who are responsible for the well-being of the mother and baby. If a teacher can become known to the hospital staffs in the area and use tact and diplomacy, mutual trust and understanding will grow. She will keep in touch with new methods and procedures and in her turn may be able to offer pointers about the home conditions and possible reactions among the parents in her groups. It may be possible to arrange that part of the course, perhaps a visit to the labour ward or a fathers' evening, is held in the hospital. One such class is described in Chapter 10.

HISTORY

Early beginnings

Since the mid-nineteenth century attempts have been made in this country to carry out various parts of these aims.

Health visitors

Preparation for the care of babies began in 1862 when the Ladies' Health Society of Manchester was formed from women who had successfully reared a family and were willing to go from house to house offering advice on, among other things, the care of children, and the feeding, washing and clothing of babies. Other towns followed Manchester's example and began to employ 'health visitors'. In 1946 the National Health Service made mothercraft classes possible all over the country and health visitors were specifically given the task of advising 'as to the care of young children and expectant and nursing mothers'. Classes spread and the content widened and altered with new understanding of the needs of pregnant women. Margaret McEwan, writing in *Health Visiting* (1957), says that 'The teaching in the past has been mainly on physical health and mothercraft. Now the importance of teaching on mental health and the importance of family relationships is fully recognised'.

It was about this time that Local Health Authorities decided to encourage 'antenatal classes for labour' in clinics, and the health visitor was ideally situated to organise these, often with a physiotherapist as colleague. In the 1950s a State Registered Nurse could not train as a health visitor without doing six months' midwifery, ending in her Part I midwifery examination. This gave her a background of obstetric knowledge, so that she could talk about events and sensations of pregnancy and labour with some authority. In fact, most health visitors at this time were also trained midwives. The requirements for training changed, and a three months' obstetric course during her SRN training is now sufficient to allow entry to the health visitor training scheme (currently one year's training). Some younger health visitors are, therefore, not quite so sure of their midwifery facts, and recently it has become routine for midwives to join them in antenatal training.

However, as Margaret McEwan foresaw, health visitors' training today concentrates much more on mental and emotional health, and the family as a unit. In their antenatal class teaching, health visitors are encouraged to discuss and explore feelings and aspirations about family life. With their experience, it is possible for them to combine classes of primiparae and multiparae, and lead group discussions which can strengthen the capacity to cope with situations after the birth of the baby. This is especially valuable for the young primiparae in the group. It helps to prepare them for the complete change of role which inevitably follows the cessation of work outside the home. The experienced mothers are asked to recall their feelings, and often describe vividly the overwhelming and sometimes claustrophobic sensations of being 'taken over' by the demands of a vociferous baby. Their experiences of a 24-hour working day, and of how it is possible to cope eventually, enable the whole group to gain confidence by shared experiences.

Group work like this enables the health visitor to become known, and be welcomed when she visits regularly after the baby's birth. Each mother knows that she will try to help her through the crises of the first months of parenthood.

Ideas about antenatal preparation for labour came somewhat later.

Physiotherapists

In 1912 Dr J. S Fairbairn was in charge of the obstetrical department of St Thomas's Hospital, London, where Miss Minnie Randell, a nurse, midwife and physiotherapist, was principal of the school of physiotherapy. They established a physical routine to restore postnatal health and began to work towards an antenatal regime which would promote physical health during pregnancy and help towards an easier labour. Margaret Morris, a professional dancer who trained as a masseuse under Miss Randell, specialised in ante- and postnatal exercises and put forward the idea that it should be possible to rehearse for labour in a way similar to that for a ballet. In 1936 she and Miss Randell published a book called *Maternal and Postnatal Exercises*. Together with Dr Kathleen Vaughan they devised talks, relaxation practice and a series of exercises to increase the flexibility of the joints of the pelvis and posture for use in labour to facilitate the descent of the baby. But Randell wrote as long ago as 1949 'the women should understand that harmonious interaction of the mind and body is essential in childbirth and that training of the muscular system goes hand in hand with training of the nervous system in order to preserve this harmony' (Randell, 1949).

Dick-Read's influence

From the 1930s onwards Dr Grantly Dick-Read exercised a great influence on antenatal education. He believed that birth in the normal woman, being a natural physiological function, should not give rise to pain. Civilisation and culture, however, have brought influences to bear upon the minds of women which mitigate against the smooth working of their natural functions and introduce fears and anxieties concerning childbirth. In labour these fears trigger off the natural protective mechanisms of the body, giving rise to tensions not only in the mind but also in the body, notably in the circular muscles of the cervix. Resistance of these muscles to normal dilatation causes pain and so more fear, hence the vicious circle of fear, tension, pain is established. Dr Dick-Read's method of alleviating fear was through wise instruction about the changes and sensations to expect in the body and an analysis of the probable changing emotional reactions culminating in the excitement and fulfilment of birth. He had very little use for any general exercise regime, but taught deep relaxation and deep slow breathing to overcome tension during the first stage of labour, followed by controlled effort during the contractions of the second stage, interspersed with relaxation between contractions. He laid great stress on the personal interest of the physician in the training and on his presence to implement it during labour.

Helen Heardman, a teacher of physiotherapy, used ideas both from the St Thomas's school and from Grantly Dick-Read. In addition to more technical books, she produced a small booklet for mothers explaining in simple terms the fear, tension, pain syndrome and suggesting methods of combating it, and this has been widely used in English-speaking countries (Ebner, 1968).

In the late 1940s Mrs Heardman called all physiotherapists interested in obstetric work together for a meeting at the Royal Free Hospital in London. The Obstetric Association of Chartered Physiotherapists was born out of this group. In their three-year training all physiotherapists are required to know the basic anatomy and physiology of the reproductive and urological systems and something of the psychological changes which may occur during puberty, pregnancy and the menopause. They are given experience in gynaecological wards and out-patients where they learn to give treatments as appropriate. In a maternity unit they watch at least one labour and give postnatal exercise classes and treatments. They watch, but do not usually take, antenatal classes. They also receive instruction in handling and, where appropriate, treating young babies.

However, obstetrics and gynaecology form a very small part of a physiotherapist's general training, and since the days of Minnie Randell and Helen Heardman it has been considered desirable that a physiotherapist who wishes to specialise in these subjects should have post-registration training. In the beginning, courses were somewhat haphazard, but in 1967 a committee was set up to re-examine the aims and activities of the Obstetric Association of Chartered Physiotherapists, conditions for membership and the content of available courses. A standard syllabus was drawn up to occupy two long weekends or five days and pilot courses were arranged in various centres in the British Isles. On March 1st 1970, all physiotherapists contemplating full membership of the association were required to attend a recognised post-registration course and to submit written evidence that they had had adequate experience of current obstetric practice during the past year.

In 1976, due largely to the work of two physiotherapists, Dorothy Mandelstam and Sheila Harrison, considerable new interest was aroused in the treatment of gynaecological conditions with particular reference to stress incontinence. The Association is indebted to them and to the wise guidance of the then President Mr John Carron Brown and later to Dame Josephine Barnes in steering the Association towards the next landmark in its history—namely, the inclusion of gynaecology in the course and the logical change of name to The Association of Chartered Physiotherapists in Obstetrics and Gynaecology.

It soon became clear that difficulties were arising in ensuring adequate supervision of prospective full members and, in some instances, of obtaining for them sufficient experience—particularly in labour and gynaecological wards. It was felt that both the syllabus and the method of assessment should be re-examined with a view to having the course recognised and validated by the Chartered Society of Physiotherapists. The country was divided into areas and a voluntary regional representative who had at least 7 years experience was appointed for each. A prospective new full member was put in touch with her representative who was to be responsible for planning her practical training and for observation and assessment of her classes. In June 1981 the new, more demanding syllabus including the observation of classes and treatments came into force.

Meanwhile work has been continuing on the preparation of a new syllabus for those wishing to qualify for full registration as an obstetric physiotherapist at an advanced level, the examination to be taken not less than 2 years after part 1. It is hoped that this qualification may one day count as a module towards a degree (Odoni, 1980). Obstetric physiotherapists are still in short supply and they have been and are being used to teach midwives and health visitors those parts of the syllabus for which they have a special expertise.

The National Childbirth Trust

The National Childbirth Trust, at first called the Natural Childbirth Association, was started in 1956 by Prunella Briance and a group of patients and admirers of Grantly Dick-Read. They felt that classes in preparation for labour were still not widely enough available, and those that were laid insufficient emphasis on pyschological preparation of parents in all aspects of childbirth. The Trust offers a meeting ground for lay and professional workers and a pressure group for more understanding care of pregnant women. Members now run a network of classes over the British Isles and train teachers. Some members have done a good deal to encourage a better understanding of childbirth among school children. Others have promoted a revival of interest and knowledge in breast feeding and the Trust is becoming known for its work in setting up postnatal support groups.

The antenatal teachers are drawn from a wide variety of backgrounds and the majority are themselves parents. A student works under the guidance of a tutor, and the training usually takes between one and two years. During this time a student attends tutorials, works through a prescribed reading list, attends a minimum of two courses taught by a qualified NCT teacher and attends two compulsory weekend seminars. In addition, the tutor will ask for some written work and suggest study events to meet the individual student's needs. Finally the student submits a teaching plan and essay for assessment by a Teachers' Panel.

On average, an antenatal course consists of eight two hour sessions which may be designed for couples or for women, with one or two classes for partners to attend. The classes are usually held in the teacher's home and groups are kept small and informal. There is almost always a reunion after all have given birth at which the teacher has an opportunity of receiving feedback from the parents.

NCT teachers aim to help both parents consider their own feelings about, and expectations of, birth and parenthood. They are trained to give up-to-date and accurate information enabling parents to understand the natural birth process, how to adapt to difficulties should they arise and to appreciate when medical intervention is necessary. Classes offer a balance between exercise, practical skills, information and discussion on the physical, practical and emotional aspects of pregnancy, labour and parenthood.

Breastfeeding counsellors also undertake a training and have all breastfed for at least three months. They talk to parents in antenatal classes and are available postnatally for support, counselling and breastfeeding advice. The postnatal network offers informal, mother to mother contact and support.

'Preparation for childbirth' classes in this country have therefore grown from two roots: parentcraft, slanted mostly towards the care of the baby, and theoretical and practical preparation for labour. In many centres good, well-integrated courses were developed and have been running for years; in others, the inspiration and enthusiasm of the pioneers had been watered down and become ineffectual. The advent of psycho-prophylaxis encouraged many people to make a new appraisal of their courses and to search for better methods of preparation and support of parents, and midwives became involved in group teaching. The 'active birth' movement seems to be inspiring new enthusiasm in both midwives and mothers.

Midwives

As their title implies, midwives are traditionally 'with the wife' in labour. Over the centuries, midwives handed their skills down, one from another, as still happens in many developing countries all over the world.

It was not until 1902 that the Midwives Act (England) set up the Central Midwives Board, to register the midwives who were practising their craft. This Board set up a recognised syllabus for the training of midwives, but this training was not compulsory until 1936, and was a practical training, with no opportunity for teaching mothers in the antenatal period. At this time, each midwife was controlled by a Local Supervisory Authority, who monitored the standards of midwives' skills and practices. Many babies were born in hospital at that time, and the head of the Authority was then an obstetrician, but many more were born at home, and the domiciliary midwives were loosely controlled by a supervisor of midwives, herself a midwife. For many years, the midwives working at home were essentially independent practitioners. During the 1940s and 1950s, some of these midwives became interested in the techniques advocated by Dr Grantly Dick Read, and started informal classes for their own patients, which were called 'relaxation' classes.

In the 1940s, training in midwifery was firmly established—a six months' training (after State Registration as a qualified nurse) in hospital would end in the First Part Midwifery certificate—trained for acting as a maternity nurse in a hospital unit, but not to work alone as a midwife. The Second Part Midwifery Certificate was gained after a further six months' training, mostly caring for women in their homes under the guidance of one or more midwives. If these midwives happened to be keen on 'relaxation' classes, the student would help in a class situation, but this was not part of the syllabus of the examination.

In the 1970s, it was considered that too many nurses were taking the Part I examination and being content with their role as maternity nurse, supervised by doctors or trained midwives, or simply using the certificate for later promotion. The course was combined as a year's full training. By this time, antenatal classes were being organised routinely both in health clinics and hospitals, and class teaching was added to the examination syllabus. Each student, in her year's training, had to participate in teaching groups of mothers in some aspect of antenatal care or labour. All these students became qualified midwives, able to act independently in normal pregnancies and labour, and also able to take their part in group teaching.

It is now firmly acknowledged, by obstetricians, that midwives are the skilled and appropriate practitioners in normal labours, and by health visitors and physiotherapists, that their expertise is valuable in class teaching.

In September 1980, the Central Midwives Board, now responsible for midwife-training in the UK, changed the midwifery training period to eighteen months for State Registered Nurses. Their basic syllabus stresses that she 'has an important contribution to make in providing health education, particularly on matters concerning parenthood, child care, the management of infant feeding, and the promotion of breast feeding.'

Under 'Health Education' the syllabus contains the following: 'Principles and methods of teaching health care, maintenance of physical and emotional wellbeing, psycho-sexual problems in relation to child-bearing, preparation for childbirth and parenthood.'

Under 'Psychology—'emotional and behavioural adaptation to pregnancy and parenthood.'

The syllabus also states that she must have practical experience in conducting parentcraft teaching sessions, under the supervision of her midwife-teacher.

Not all midwives will wish to continue group teaching, but certainly the ones who are keen to do so are now being prepared for it during their training.

As will be seen by the above, health visitors, midwives and obstetric physiotherapists are all being trained for antenatal teaching. To avoid conflict, the Health Visitors' Association and the Royal College of Midwives issued a joint statement in 1982.

The paragraph in the statement which is applicable to this book reads as follows:

'The midwife and health visitor both have responsibilities for health education in the antenatal period. There will need to be discussion between them to decide how they can best contribute to the antenatal classes.

All antenatal education should be designed to provide not only neccessary information and advice but also an opportunity for both prospective parents to express and discuss all their needs, fears and expectations.

The syllabus should include, as a minimum, information about:

Pregnancy, labour and delivery—   Given by a midwife.

Infant feeding
Diet
Family planning   Given by midwives and health visitors
Fetal development
Care of the infant
Family relationships

Midwives and health visitors are working closely with obstetric physiotherapists whenever possible.

Other valuable contributors, when appropriate and available, could include—anaesthetists, dentists, dietitians, obstetricians, paediatricians, and social workers. These additional contributors and variations in the syllabus will be influenced by local needs and factors.

Hypnosis

During the 1940s observations were being made in England and some European countries, particularly in Russia, of the effects of hypnosis in childbirth, and favourable results in the suppression of pain were achieved. However, this method was not applicable to large numbers, and had certain other disadvantages. In 1949, Velvovski, a neuropsychiatrist, and some of his obstetrical colleagues described a new method which they called 'psycho-prophylaxis', which attempted to overcome the disadvantages of hypnosis by offering a form of active mental preparation to groups of women.

Psychoprophylaxis

This method was based on the concept that reflex actions of the body can be conditioned by differing stimuli. Pavlov demonstrated that dogs, conditioned to expect food by the ringing of a bell at the same time as food was presented to them, would soon salivate at the sound of the bell, even if they could neither see nor smell food. Velvovsky and his colleagues put forward the idea that the childbearing woman was conditioned by hearsay to associate labour with pain, therefore when she experienced any new sensation from her uterus in labour, these sensations were signalled to the brain and immediately interpreted as those of pain. They set out to 'decondition' these harmful verbal associations by education about normal pregnancy and birth and by constant assurance that 'labour pain is not an inborn attribute of women or an inalienable element of normal childbirth' (Velvovsky et al., 1960).

Another principle of the preparation was the use of activity to raise the pain threshold. Patients were taught to associate special kinds of breathing and self-massage with the onset of contractions, and they found that, in labour, these 'useful stimuli' were often strong enough to cut out painful stimuli. The women were taught that the human brain responds to messages like a complicated telephone switchboard, which can only handle a certain number of incoming and outgoing messages at once and will register preferentially the ones considered most important, blocking others which would distract or interfere. The teaching had to be precise, and the women had to practise daily what was taught in class to build up the habit of the 'correct response', and to be able to concentrate on that response to block painful sensations.

In 1951, Dr Fernand Lamaze, of the Clinique des Metallurgistes in Paris, visited Russia and was very impressed by what he saw of this new teaching, named 'psychoprophylaxis' or 'mind prevention'. He began to use the techniques in his own clinic, and soon his methods were discussed throughout France, where they were called 'accouchement sans douleur'. Lamaze taught different kinds of response to uterine contractions, namely, rapid shallow breathing over the height of late first stage contractions to prevent diaphragmatic pressure on the uterus, and a form of localised relaxation which he called 'decontraction', to prevent other muscles, particularly those of the abdominal wall and pelvic floor, contracting in association with those of the uterus.

Doctors, midwives, physiotherapists and health visitors from many parts of the world visited the Clinique des Metallurgistes and observed the work of Lamaze and later of his associates Vellay and Hersilie. Some, like Erna Wright who at that time was teaching at the National Childbirth Trust, accepted the whole doctrine and set out to spread it by means of lectures, seminars, and a popular book *The New Childbirth*, others used parts of the method and built it into their own. Such a mixture is anathema to the purists but some major differences already seem to have arisen between different schools of psychoprophylaxis; for example, the French still insist on the validity of the title 'accouchement sans douleur' while the Russians have 'considered it wiser not to stress the pain factor in the new nomenclature' (Chertok, 1959).

Many proponents of psychoprophylaxis, though paying tribute to Dick-Read, believe that their method is completely new and different. They say that Pavlovian explanations of cortical conditioning offer a much more scientific explanation than Read's 'fear, tension, pain' theory, and that 'he gives the woman a passive role through dilatation while psychoprophylaxis gives her as much activity as possible throughout labour' (Vellay, 1959). Dick-Read stressed the time and patience required by the physician conducting a 'natural childbirth'. Heardman or one of her associates was present at most of the labours of her trained mothers. Vellay uses professional 'monitrices', and other obstetricians train fathers to act as 'labour coaches'. The Russians and others have tried to secure informed support for their prepared mothers by training courses, not just for those responsible for the preparation, but for the *whole* staff of the unit, lasting in the case of doctors for as long as three months. It is this involvement and enthusiasm of *all* who work with the parents that seems to characterise successful labour preparation; Lee Buxton (1962), an American obstetrician who spent a year studying various methods of psychosomatic preparation, remarks that he finds this of more importance than differences in methodology.

It should be noted that psychoprophylaxis is essentially a preparation for labour, and stops short at the moment of delivery; postnatal rehabilitation of the mother and care of the baby are not considered to be part of the course. 'Puériculture' in France is either a completely separate antenatal course, or classes are held in the maternity hospitals immediately after confinement. In England, owing to the increasing tendency towards early discharge and to pressure of work in many maternity units, attempts are being made to put more emphasis on this aspect, particularly on the mental health side, into the antenatal classes.

Later developments

Another development, common to other forms of education, which has been marked during the last few years has been a move away from authoritarian teaching to a much greater involvement of the group as a whole. Members are encouraged to discuss their feelings, to evaluate their attitudes, and to make up their own minds about their actions, providing these do not conflict with their own or their babies' safety. This trend has been encouraged by the influence of parents associations such as the National Childbirth Trust in the British Isles, the International Childbirth Education Association in the United States and the Parents' Federation of New Zealand, and by such teachers as the social anthropologist, Sheila Kitzinger (1972).

Active birth

More recently, there has been a further move away from the teaching of 'psychoprophylaxis'. Rigid breathing patterns and 'mind-blocking' techniques have been replaced by encouragement to mothers to keep mobile, to find their own positions of comfort, and to behave 'instinctively' during contractions. Two prominent obstetricians in this field have been Dr R. Caldeyro-Barcia in Montevideo, and Dr Michel Odent in Pithiviers, France. While Dr Odent has invited people to observe his methods, both at his unit and on film, Dr Caldeyro-Barcia has produced statistical evidence that active, ambulant women have shorter labours with more effective contractions.

Nevertheless, we cannot leave everything to 'instinct'. The mothers in the above units were guided antenatally and in labour by experienced attendants, and had been taught the processes of labour. Without some knowledge of the happenings in labour, and how to relax muscles and 'let the body work', there is a danger that the instinctive behaviour would be the 'fight or flight' reflex which Grantly Dick Read campaigned against. With knowledge, however, and the ability to find comfortable positions, a woman may indeed be better to remain active in the first stage of labour, with gravity helping the descent of the baby's head and aiding dilatation of the cervix.

Perhaps we are re-learning what Minnie Randell taught, and today her *Training for Childbirth* (1949) looks very modern, with similar positions to those in Dr Odent's *Salle Sauvage* in Pithiviers. There, the woman is encouraged to concentrate on the sensations coming from the uterus, to understand and harmonise with them, and to live through them as an experience. So that she can be completely mobile, no drugs are used—indeed, rather than medication in a difficult labour, Dr Odent prefers a Caesarian section. Because of the confidence and support throughout the unit, the mothers do manage without drugs, and the Caesarian rate is low.

Some maternity units in this country are now encouraging mobility, especially in the first stage of labour, with comfortable chairs and special beds, in attractively decorated 'birthing rooms', replacing some traditional labour wards. The most important need in labour, however, is an attendant who will support a mother and help her to harmonise with the sensations of her body.

Classes for both parents

A further development, begun in America by organisations such as the New York Maternity Center, and individuals, notably Dr Robert A. Bradley, of Denver, Colorado, has been to encourage husbands to attend not one or two 'special' classes arranged for them, but to be deeply involved in the whole course of teaching. This means that, throughout the course, they are learning with their wives, and practising ways to support and help them in labour. Many classes have now been started in this country on similar lines and are proving to be successful. Some suggestions for the organisation of such classes will be found in Chapter 10. It means, of course, that both the teacher and the couples have to be prepared to give up evenings for this, and one can imagine that a teacher with, for instance, a busy family life and small children, could find it difficult to do so. Husbands also may be tired at the end of the day. The most successful classes seem to be those in which very experienced teachers have the confidence to integrate husbands/partners completely into the class situation. The people who are now involved in this type of class say that it is not difficult when one husband, for instance, cannot arrive at a class: another husband simply helps two women instead of one, quite naturally and easily.

Classes for multigravidae

Another type of very informal class, which we would recommend, is a shortened course, or even one class, for multiparae who have previously attended a full course of classes. These 'refresher' classes, which can be found in many different parts of the country, are essentially to reinforce previous training. They provide reminders, reassurance and encouragement to mothers who have had varied experiences of labour, and who want to feel more 'in control' of their bodies in their next labours. The classes can be held in a clinic or health centre, or in a room attached to a functioning antenatal clinic, whether in hospital or in a GP's surgery. Perhaps the most successful are in the home of the teacher, or of one of the group. If a daytime class is planned, it is essential that 'minders' are found for the other children. If children in class do not distract the rest of the group they certainly occupy the mother, so that she cannot become a true participant in the session. It is preferable that the group is small—perhaps four to six people would be ideal—and open-ended, so that time can be spent in sharing previous experiences and present expectations.

Because maternity units are changing, discussion of recent developments and modern trends is a major part of this type of class, together with reminders of relaxation and breathing techniques, and help in conquering previous difficulties. A major change in some maternity hospitals has been not only to allow more movement during the first stage of labour, but to actively encourage mobility. Many women, when encouraged to move, find that gentle pelvic rocking, perhaps while on hands and knees, or when sitting in different positions, makes contractions a great deal more comfortable. Multiparae need to be taught these movements, so that they can use them if they wish, instead of lying passively for long periods, which they may have been taught previously and accepted as the routine during labour.

Often, the teacher will find, in these small groups, that she can remain in the background, while the mothers share experiences and help each other.

Pre-conceptual care

One kind of pre-conceptual care has been practised for a long time—this is the guidance and advice given to a couple who have already had difficulties. These may be of subfertility, early abortion, stillbirth, or the birth of a damaged child.

In these cases, the obstetrician and/or geneticist will be treating and testing the couple as patients. There may be hormonal or chromosomal investigations, and advice about statistical chances of inherited defects. Recently, series of controlled trials on mothers who have delivered children suffering from spina bifida have been carried out. These seem to show that extra iron and folic acid in very early pregnancy in these mothers reduces the chance of the birth of a further spina bifida baby to a significant degree, and a theory is being formed that malabsorbtion of these substances may be one of the causes of this deformity. There is as yet no proof, however, that if all women took extra iron and folic acid, no babies suffering from spina bifida and hydrocephalus would be born. Specialist medical advice will continue to be available, and further research will continue, to help these groups.

Recently, however, there has been a campaign for 'pre-conceptual care' for all, largely spearheaded by Margaret and Arthur Wynn, after the publication of their book *The Prevention of Handicap of Early Pregnancy Origin*. An organisation, Foresight, now publishes guidelines for future parents, which include the following:

Stopping oral contraception at least three months before becoming pregnant

Avoiding cigarettes, alcohol and drugs

Fresh air, exercise, and a healthy toned body

Special advice on diet, with emphasis on wholefoods, unadulterated foods, fresh fruit and vegetables, and vitamins

They also recommend hair analysis to detect lead and other metals, and harmful minerals in the body

Any pioneer organisation has to be wholehearted in its approach to attract attention, and their dedication and devotion to healthy living will no doubt be followed by many women, especially those who are already interested in health foods, yoga and positive health.

But what about the average woman, especially the one expecting her first baby?

The Wynns show clearly that statistically it is the poor and unfit whose babies are less healthy, and these are the ones who are more likely to have an unpremeditated pregnancy. How do we reach them?

Some ideas:

1. Much more linking of health and pregnancy in schools. Teenage girls are interested in pregnancy, and the following classes could be linked with a fit body, ready for pregnancy whenever it occurs:

   P. E. classes

   Classes on smoking, alcohol, drugs, contraception

   Home economics and nutrition.

2. Family planning clinics could help much more in planned pregnancies. One of us works in a clinic where patients are encouraged to return to the family planning clinic when planning a pregnancy. They are taught 'safe' methods of birth control when waiting the three months after stopping the contraceptive pill, encouraged to reach a reasonably 'ideal' weight, and given a leaflet on exercise, good eating, and advice about smoking and drinking. These patients are motivated, and have the leaflet at home to remind them of the aim of positive health before pregnancy is achieved.

3. General practitioners are becoming interested in giving pre-pregnancy advice, and at least one (Moxon, 1982) has organised a pre-conceptual counselling clinic in his practice.
4. In second and subsequent pregnancies, the mothers are in touch with their health visitors, and often discuss the timing or spacing of future pregnancies. A health visitor's role is primarily health education, and she can, on a one-to-one basis, teach pre-conceptual care.
5. In some areas, health visitors are already organising pre-conceptual clinics on a regular basis. When these are known, and discussed, the general population round these clinics will become more aware of the concept of good health *before* pregnancy.

A reasonable degree of physical fitness and an acceptable height:weight ratio is desirable when planning a pregnancy since this will involve extra activity for all the systems of the body. Ideally, this should be carried through from early childhood—squatting and kneeling are natural postures for a young child and are usually encouraged in later physical education classes, but control of the pelvic floor muscles for girls is rarely taught in schools and could be of great value. Activities and games are popular at school, but the ability to relax is less common and would be of great value to men as well as to women whatever their life style. When they leave school, girls have other interests and are apt to regard physical activities as childish, or they marry young and are too busy with a job and a home to do any routine toning up exercises.

For anybody wishing to start a baby, regular walking, swimming or jogging with a weekly session of dancing, yoga or a Keep Fit class would lay a good foundation. Women with one or more children are in a different position since they usually get plenty of activity (though it may not necessarily include full range body movement or training for the lungs and heart). Their problem is to get enough rest.

REFERENCES

Buxton, L. (1962) *A Study of Psychophysical Methods for Relief of Childbirth.* Philadelphia: Saunders.

Central Midwives Board. (1980) *Approved Midwifery Training Syllabus.*

Chertok, L. (1959) *Psychosomatic Methods in Painless Childbirth.* p. 164. Oxford: Pergamon.

Health Visitors' Association. (1982) Joint Statement on Ante-Natal Preparation. The Royal College of Midwives.

Kitzinger, S. (1972) *The Experience of Childbirth*, 3rd edition. Harmondsworth: Penguin.

Kitzinger, S. (1977) *Education and Counselling for Childbirth.* London: Baillière Tindall.

McEwan, M. (1957) *Health Visiting*, p. 109. London: Faber & Faber.
Moxon P. (1982) Caring for baby when it's only just been thought of. *Medical News*, **14**: 30, 28–29
Odoni, J. (1980) A.C.P.O.G. up-to-date. *Newsletter of Association of Chartered Physiotherapists in Obstetrics and Gynecology*, 15–18.
Randell, M. (1949) *Training for Childbirth*, 4th edition, page 45. London: Churchill.
Vellay, P. (1959) *Childbirth without Pain*, p. 3. London: Allen & Unwin.
Velvovsky, I., Platanov, K., Ploticher, V. & Shugom, E. (1960) *Painless Childbirth Through Psychoprophylaxis*. Moscow: Foreign Languages Publishing House.

FOR FURTHER READING

Caldeyro-Barcia, R. (1980) Physiological and psychological bases for the modern and humanised management of normal labour. *Scientific Publication No. 858 of the Latin-American Center of Perinatology and Human Development, Montevideo, Uruguay*. Washington: World Health Organization.
Caldeyro-Barcia, R. (1981) *The Physiological Bases for a Modern and Humanised Obstetrics*. London: National Childbirth Trust.
Davis, Adele (1978) *Let's Have Healthy Children*. London: Unwin Paperback.
Davis, E. (1981) *A Guide to Midwifery: Heart and Hands*. New Mexico: John Muir Publications.
Dickerson, J. W. T., Baker, S., Barnes, B. (1980) *Environmental Factors and Foetal Health—the Case for Pre-Conceptual Care*. Godalming, Surrey: Foresight.
Perkins, E. R. & Morris, B. (1979) Preparation for parenthood: A critique of the concept. *Leverhulme Health Education Project*. Nottingham: University of Nottingham.
Ebner, M. (1982) *Relaxation and Exercise for Natural Childbirth*, 5th edition. Edinburgh: Churchill Livingstone.
Ebner, M. (1973) *A Way to Natural Childbirth*, 3rd edition. Edinburgh: Churchill Livingstone.
Lamaze, F. (1958) *Painless Childbirth—Psychoprophylactic Techniques*. London: Burke.
Le Fanu, J. Scientific support for natural childbirth claims. *Medical News*, **14**: 13, 10
McLeary, G. F. (1935) *The Maternity and Child Welfare Movement*. London: Staples. Out of print but available from reference libraries.
Nixon, W. C. W. (1962) *Childbirth*. Harmondsworth: Penguin.
Perkins, E. R. & Morris, B. (1979) Preparation for parenthood: A critique of the concept. *Leverhulme Health Education Project*. Nottingham: University of Nottingham.
Odent, M. (1981) *Genese De L'Homme Ecologique* Newsletter 14. London: Birth Centre.
Odent, M. (1981) *Birth at Pithiviers* Newsletter 16. London: Birth Centre.
Gillett, J. R. (1979) Childbirth in Pithiviers, France. *Lancet*, **2**, 894–896.
Pickard, B. M. (1981) *Are you Fit Enough to become Pregnant?* Leeds: Pickard, The University of Leeds. Available NCT.
Pickard, B. (1982) *Be Fit and Healthy Before You Start a Baby*. Pickard, Lane End Farm, Denton, Ilkley, West Yorks.
Snaith, L. & Coxon, A. (1968) Dick-Read's *Childbirth Without Fear*, 5th edition. London: Heinemann.
Wright, E. (1964) *The New Childbirth*. London: Tandem.
Wynn A. & M. (1979) *The Prevention of Handicap of Early Pregnancy Origin*. London: The Foundation for Children and Research into Childbearing.

2

Teaching techniques

Teaching is a form of communication. The techniques that we use are therefore all designed to achieve understanding between ourselves and the members of our classes, whether we are describing the course of labour, trying to help a woman to explore the way her body works, or discussing her feelings towards her baby. When planning a course we need to define its purpose, consider its content, organise the material, decide on the mode of presentation, and evaluate the results (Beard, 1970).

The broad aims of antenatal education were discussed in the previous chapter. When further defining their purpose we need to break down each of these aims into smaller teaching projects, then think clearly how we can 'put over' each of these. This is not a once and for all decision, but the questions we set ourselves and the answers we find will change continually as our understanding of parents' needs increases. It is, however, fatally easy to accept some part of another teacher's programme and incorporate it into one's own, without applying the aims test sufficiently carefully. This is particularly true of exercises—one watches an attractive exercise and one is apt to try it out on a class without thinking exactly what it is supposed to do.

The use of different techniques

At present it seems that the needs we have stated are best met in three ways: by talks, discussion, and physical education. Different teachers may specialise in any one of these techniques but the triangle should have approximately equal sides as far as the time spent on each aspect is concerned.

We are lucky that most of our mothers, though perhaps fewer of their partners, are highly motivated towards classes and are therefore a very receptive group. On the other hand, we may have in the groups individuals with widely differing educational and cultural backgrounds, and must somehow stimulate and hold the interest of

21

each one of them. Research indicates that if intelligent or educated patients are to follow advice they need a non-patronising non-directive approach, with plenty of information, which is not one-sided and over optimistic. On the other hand, less well educated patients will respond better with a simpler more directive approach with less information; however, the information provided should be specific and stressed as very important (Wagstaff, 1982). This applies particularly to exercises and postures which one wants to encourage mothers to practise. The attention span even of a university student at a lecture is said to be not longer than 20 minutes. In our classes it may well be no more than 10 minutes, but we can remain in communication longer if we teach our students through their eyes, hands and bodies as well as through their ears. A wise educational maxim says, 'I hear and I forget, I see and I remember, I do and I understand'. The attention of a class has a wave-like form—it starts high, wanes, then recovers, so that it is a good idea to put the most important points at the beginning and end of the talk. Even in an informal teaching situation, where questions and discussions are encouraged during a talk, there must be a framework of order, otherwise the teacher finds that important points have been left out and the class is not clear what it has learned. One is reminded of the negro preacher who on being asked how he was able to attract such large congregations replied, 'I tells 'em what I goin' to tell 'em, I tells 'em, then I tells 'em what I told 'em'.

TALKS

Organisation of material

If one is planning a course it is tremendously helpful to spend some time listening to similar classes given by an experienced teacher, not only to hear what subjects she chooses and how she 'puts them over' but also to observe reactions in the audience, what catches their interest, what makes them fidget, what questions they ask. Having planned the subjects for one's own talks one must keep in touch with modern developments, whether this involves reading the latest catalogue of maternity wear and baby equipment or visiting the labour wards. If one is working outside hospital then it is essential to visit those units which members of the class will attend, getting to know the staffs and be known by them, and keeping informed about the latest procedures. One must also attend meetings and read widely around the subjects, not only in up-to-date textbooks but in the popular press, and watch relevant broadcast programmes since it is these which will stimulate questions. It is said that a lecture is like an iceberg, the seventh part which is above the water is actually used in the talk, the remaining six-sevenths is below and is the background information which may be uncovered by questions and discussion.

Suppose the subject for the first talk is to be the changes of early pregnancy; the material is carefully selected and sifted, remembering always that we are not trying to train medical students nor midwives but to help a mother through the experience of pregnancy, so that everything must be relevant to *her* baby, *her* body, *her* sensations and *her* emotions. For example, a long dissertation, actually overheard at a recent class, on the exact methods of transfer of nutritive substances by diffusion through the walls of the chorionic villi in the placenta, obviously bored the women to tears, but a discussion of the foods to eat which would keep their babies healthy would have held their interest.

Choice of words

Words and images must be chosen with great care. One is between the Scylla of a too technical presentation and the Charybdis of talking down to one's audience. If, as so often happens, the teacher is a woman, the group will identify with her more readily if she talks about '*our* bodies behaving in such a way' rather than '*your* bodies'. It is important to include some medical terms because the women will overhear these in clinics and hospitals and may puzzle over them. Also, knowledge of the right words gives them a pleasant feeling of competence and will stand them in good stead when they come to educate their own children. However, it is better not to presuppose knowledge, and terms like uterus and placenta should always be prefixed by the lay terms womb and afterbirth. One must also remember that some common midwifery expressions can be frightening to lay people: for example, a woman was reduced to tears by overhearing two students say that her baby's head was still 'free'.

Verbal pictures can be very helpful, but they must always relate the unknown to the known, the simile of the baby fitting into the pelvis like an egg into an egg cup is meaningful to most people, but the description of coping with a contraction like riding a wave on a surfboard is not going to mean anything to a group of Indian women who have rarely seen the sea. A knowledge of the cultural background, and ideas about childbirth current in the community from which the mothers come is therefore essential, and a readiness to change images if one is met with a blank stare. Examples taken from personal or professional experience enliven a talk, particularly if these are spiced with a type of humour which is acceptable to the group.

Preparing the talk

Having prepared the material, and thought out the images and examples, beginners will find it helpful to write the talk out in full and, in a room alone, read it over fairly slowly, timing the length in two or three readings. If a tape recorder is available this is an excellent way of judging the effectiveness of the talk, and correcting any irritating voice mannerisms. When the content is reasonably well known, key words or phrases are underlined in red. When reading through the next time, the eye should try to focus only on the underlined words, getting the flow of the rest from memory, and not attempting to recreate the speech exactly as written. The underlined words can be transferred to a small card, and the talk again rehearsed. The small card is then the only 'memory tool' necessary. To give confidence, the first sentence of the talk can be written at the top of the card, but with sufficient rehearsal, even a diffident speaker can give an interesting talk, if she herself feels the subject to be important and meaningful. It will soon become possible to give the talk from memory, then the problem arises of introducing subtle changes to make it sound fresh and spontaneous.

Another method is to jot down headings as they occur to one, put them in order, then talk to oneself about them, trying out various ways of expressing the points, finally noting sufficient words or phrases to recall the flow of the talk. This has the advantage that the ideas are expressed in spoken rather than written English from the beginning. There is a lot to be said for letting a talk lie fallow in one's subconscious mind for several days and trying out the occasional phrase, perhaps while doing something quite irrelevant, before committing anything to paper. Appropriate audiovisual aids (see Ch. 3) are then chosen and put ready. Alternatively, if the talk is a commentary on a series of slides or a film it is better to project these and build up the verbal explanations around them.

Presentation

All are frightened the first time they have to speak in public no matter whether they are going to deliver an hour's lecture or spend one minute proposing the acceptance of a report. They feel that they may be exposing themselves to ridicule, aggression, or even humiliation, like a child that has annoyed its parents. Even the experienced speaker is slightly nervous before giving a talk, particularly if the subject or type of audience is not his usual one. Some degree of nervousness should be welcomed since it stimulates adrenaline production, makes the speaker more alive and interesting, and increases her sensitivity and therefore her communication with her audience. Lucky people cut their teeth (or perhaps 'grow their speaker's tongues' would be a better metaphor) in some informal committee, but others may suddenly be told that they must give a talk on a certain subject to a selected group on a certain date. The answer lies in meticulous preparation and it is hoped that the early part of this chapter may be helpful.

Further preparations

Some further preparations of the room are needed just before the class assembles (see Ch. 4). It may be necessary for the teacher to wear uniform, but ordinary dress creates much less of a barrier between herself and her audience, particularly if it is quiet in colour and style but sufficiently up to date to give confidence among a group of critical young women. Slacks, or tights and a loose skirt, are essential if the teacher is also going to teach exercises, but, even if she is not, she will often need plenty of freedom to move, for example to demonstrate the bony points of the pelvis on her body. Face and hair should be checked before entering the room and then can be forgotten.

Self-confidence and complete ease of manner only come with practice, but given a knowledge of the subject and a real interest in the audience, not just in their medical histories, but in themselves as women, most speakers can make a 'good job' even of their first classes. As the teacher's confidence grows so will that of the group. The essential factors are a belief in the value of what one is talking about, and a deep interest in the problems and joys of young parents. In our opinion teachers without this enthusiasm should never be asked to take antenatal classes; the people in them are far too sensitive to atmosphere.

Use of the voice

How then do you express this interest and enthusiasm? First, you use your voice to its best advantage so that you sound as if you find the whole subject fascinating. It is to be hoped that you have already practised with a tape recorder or on long-suffering colleagues so that you know that your voice is well modulated, neither too quick nor too slow, too low nor too high, and is free from 'ers and ums'. Verbal punctuation is important, a pause between sentences, a change of speed, or stress on one particular word, all add to the interest of a talk. A great deal can be learned by listening to actors on television or in the theatre with these points in mind. Some amateur dramatic training is a great help to an antenatal teacher and even such exercises as stressing different words in a sentence and noticing the differing meanings which result can be helpful. Try stressing in turn each of the words in the following sentence: 'I never said he stole that purse'.

Non-verbal communication

To express and generate interest you must also remember that you are not just talking *at* people but trying to communicate with them. It is very easy to fix your eyes on your notes or on some particular member of the class who seems sympathetic, resulting in the rest of the class feeling left out and the unfortunate recipient of your glance wondering if a bra strap is showing. So, you turn your head, looking from person to person so that everybody feels she is important; note the general reaction. Do they look interested or are they asleep, fidgeting or yawning? If so, can you make a change, show an interesting picture, ask a question, try out an exercise? After experimenting for a bit it can be very helpful to ask a colleague to sit in on a class and make honest comments, particularly about any irritating mannerisms of which you may be quite unconscious. A few months ago one of us was in this situation and was asked if she knew that she crossed one leg over the other very firmly every time she came to a vital bit of her discourse.

Questions

One of the tests of a good class is the number and variation of the questions put, and the amount of discussion which arises. It is usually best to encourage people to ask questions as soon as they occur to them, to watch for the puzzled frown or the mouth half opened to comment and, indeed, it is a good idea to pause frequently to ask 'is that clear?' or 'would anybody like to say something about this point?' If the thread of the talk is temporarily broken one can always ask the women to recall the last point, so encouraging feed-back from them. Usually, no question asked in class is academic; the woman has some personal reason for asking, and one must be careful not to answer in a facile or quick manner, but to try to see any other meaning behind the question. For example, a woman in class asked how long was the umbilical cord. I could have said 'about 46 to 71 cm (18 to 28 inches)' and passed on, but I then asked how many had heard the nonsensical old wives' tale of the cord getting round the baby's neck if a woman put her hands above her head, continuing with the reassurance that, if the baby happened to get the cord round his neck, the midwives had a simple technique to deal with this after the birth of the head. A discussion of other old wives' tales followed, with the class seeming enormously relieved to get them explained, and to know that most of them had been some-what worried and half-believing, even of the oddest tales. Later, the woman who had asked the original question said that her grand-mother had seen her hanging out clothes, and had told her she would strangle her baby by doing so. This is a simple illustration, but serves to warn all teachers to be sensitive when dealing with any question, and explore for the hidden question behind the one which is asked. Nobody is omniscient and there will certainly be questions which I cannot answer; I admit it freely, promise to find out and *keep* that promise the following week.

INDIVIDUAL COUNSELLING

Even in the most relaxed class, some women prefer to ask their ques-tions when alone with the teacher, and she should make herself unobtrusively available before and after class and during coffee or tea breaks. She should also be prepared to suggest a time when she would be free for a longer private chat with one or both parents, either in a small room or on the telephone. The request for a private talk may come from the teacher herself if she thinks that may be helpful to a woman who seems worried. In these circumstances it is so easy to jump in with advice or an explanation that we think will allay fear, much more difficult to keep silent and listen. Listening has truly been called the lost art of this age. One needs not just to recognise the sounds that come out of another person's mouth but to try to understand the meaning that underlies her particular choice of words, her hesitations and gestures. One should realise the prejudices which these words may be arousing in oneself and suspend judgement until the other person's point of view is thoroughly expressed. It may help to put a question, such as 'Do you mean that?' or show one's attention by rephrasing a sentence and asking, 'Have I got this clear?' but basically one's function is to be a sympathetic listener.

Some teachers make an individual interview with one or preferably both parents part of their course. This may be the only way to help a foreigner who has little command of English. Sometimes the husband or a friend can act as interpreter, and most of the teaching has to be done visually and through touch. For example, the teacher can demonstrate relaxation with her own body.

There are other opportunities for useful one-to-one teaching, for example, those afforded by home visits by midwives and health visitors, and later by midwives in the early phases of labour. It is also possible to teach basic relaxation and control in early labour, with a description of what is happening. This is tremendously valuable with a nervous mother who has not been to classes. One of us (M. W.) pays regular visits to a hospital antenatal ward when it is often possible to arouse interest in multiparous women and unmarried primipara who might otherwise not come to classes. The other (D. B.) finds individual teaching in the home is accepted well and absorbed. The home teaching may be very necessary especially with immigrant women who are not used to leaving the house. It is valuable if the interpreter, when needed, is her husband, as he then sees he also can have a role to play in labour.

GROUP DISCUSSION

Human beings are sociable animals. Each of us belongs to a number of groups and interacts in different ways with other members of these groups. To quote Klein (1961) 'The individual needs his groups' assurance that he is valued, he gains it by behaving in a manner acceptable to the group; and when he does this he gives to others the same assurance of individual worth which he gains from them'. When women become pregnant, especially when that pregnancy becomes obvious to others and it is a first pregnancy, they often feel the need for membership of the new group. They are no longer carefree young lovers but are continually reminded of coming responsibilities which their friends may not yet have undertaken. Particularly if the couple have recently moved, the parentcraft class may supply the friends and support which they need. They may join the class in search of information from the teacher, but stay because they look forward to exchanging ideas and experiences with the rest of the group, who have a tremendously strong bond of interest.

Listening to a talk can be a completely passive learning experience—indeed, it can flow over an audience leaving little behind, but involvement in a discussion is active and encourages thought. Group members will often enlarge upon or reinforce the teacher's experiences using different words which will be remembered. There is a consensus of opinion among educationalists that discussion is better than formal teaching for changing attitudes. Problems which might be embarrassing in a two-person relationship can be discussed very generally in a group, and no one need feel that she is under attack since no one needs to acknowledge that the problem is hers. Members of a group are comforted when some problem they had thought peculiar to themselves is brought to light and proves to be quite a common experience. This aspect can be particularly helpful to the shy woman who finds it difficult to ask questions or express her feelings. Some women are relieved to hear about another's worry which does not bother them, and take pleasure in supporting the worried member of the group.

From the leader's point of view, group discussion is a fascinating but far from easy method of teaching, for it involves the teacher in a change of role. 'She deliberately withdraws from being the focus of attention, and her efforts are directed towards encouraging interaction among all the members, this includes herself but not as the dominating member' (Abercrombie, 1970). She can find out how much the group knows and whether the information has been given at approximately the right speed and depth. She can observe the interaction within the group, and may be alerted to some particular difficulty or problem; for example, an undesirable attitude towards some other member of the antenatal team or ambivalence towards the coming baby.

Preparation of material

Discussion may start spontaneously at any time during the class, and one of the benefits which arises from the type of class that we have been describing is that time is always allowed for it. On the other hand, it may be desirable to base the discussion on a prepared talk, filmstrip or film. Other ways of giving impetus to a discussion are to invite a previous member of the class to come back for a visit with her baby, to read a labour report from an ex-class member, to listen to a tape or record or to ask a thought-provoking question. 'With what do you associate the word pain?' is a good way of starting an interesting interchange of ideas on that subject. Whatever way is chosen, the group leader must think carefully about her introduction and read around the relevant facts. She should be familiar with any material that is presented, including the labour reports, so that she can explain and discuss any difficulties that may have arisen.

Management

The group of perhaps 5 to 15 is best arranged in a compact circle; the participants either sit on chairs or on cushions on the floor with their backs comfortably supported against the walls, close enough together so that gestures and expressions are easily visible. Research has shown that the leader is more readily accepted as a member of the group if her chair or cushions are exactly the same as those of the class, and equidistant from the others. She may answer factual questions, but must remember that the object is not a dialogue between herself and one member of the group but an interchange of views between different members, so that the less she speaks the better. An expression of opinion can be 'batted' around with 'What do the rest of you think about this?' or even 'How do you feel about that one, Mrs.J.?' It is very helpful to have several people in the group who are already parents; if there are no multigravid women, then visitors, colleagues, even projectionists can be involved and the women pregnant for the first time will have mothers, sisters and friends who have talked about their pregnancies. It is especially valuable if mothers and fathers who have been to classes return with their babies and talk about their experiences.

The leader should greet each contribution with a smile or a glance, to express approval. It is surprising how even experienced group leaders sometimes show more approval towards one participant, and one knows how damaging this can be to the others' self-esteem. The object is to involve as many people as possible, and the shy can sometimes be encouraged to speak by a skilfully timed open-ended question, that is, one that asks for an expression of opinion rather than a yes or no; but in our opinion if people do not wish to speak they should be left in peace, and they may well talk things over with their husbands when they get home. It is difficult for the new group leader to tolerate silence, she tends to become tense herself and to pour out a stream of questions or information. To quote Sheila Kitzinger, 'Sometimes the comments that arise following a period of silence in a relaxed atmosphere, the half-expressed thoughts, the introduction of a query, the recounting of a dream or something that somebody has said that has been on her mind, can lead to a much deeper perceptiveness on the part of the leader'.

Keeping control

Fortunately there is rarely any difficulty in persuading groups of expectant parents to talk. The opposite is more often the case: how to get them to stop. If the group members wander along side paths they should be allowed to go if this is obviously proving therapeutic to them, even if it means omitting some of the points the leader intended to raise; she can make a note of these, raise them later or add them to the next talk. Some discipline is required, though it must be of the 'iron hand in the velvet glove' variety. One woman must not be allowed to monopolise the group—the woman who cannot resist the telling of horror stories is a case in point; if a change of subject or a glance does not stop her, then it can be suggested that she might like to come and talk things over with the leader privately. Nor must the group be allowed to splinter so that several different conversations are going on at the same time; these can be left for the tea break. Finally, it is better to disperse the members of a group while they are feeling alert and talkative and will go on with the conversation while they are changing or walking home rather than prolong the discussion until they are dull and 'talked out'. Before saying goodbye, it is often helpful to sum up the different viewpoints if these have been controversial, or, if not, to give the consensus of opinion so that participants can think it over during the week.

NEUROMUSCULAR CONTROL

We have now considered two sides of the preparation for childbirth triangle—talks and discussion—the third side of which is the teaching of neuromuscular control. This lengthy synonym has been chosen advisedly instead of the simpler term 'exercises' because the intention is *not* simply to give the mothers a series of movements once a week but to build up their 'body awareness' by a progressive scheme of training extending over the full course with much encouragement to practise at home. We are trying to improve their sensitivity to incoming messages from their skin, muscles and joints, to code them and to send out appropriate replies. For example, the balance of the body changes considerably during pregnancy and unless a woman is made aware of this and helped to realign her spine she leans further and further back until she achieves the true 'drummer boy' posture.

Relaxation

There are many methods of teaching relaxation, and most teachers find that they need to adapt their methods to suit different couples: what works for one pair is less successful for another.

Some teachers, like Jane Madders (1980), use touch relaxation—they ask the parents to work in pairs with one tightening and relaxing a large muscle, such as the biceps, while the other one grips the upper arm and actually feels the hardening and slackening of the muscle. Having learned the sensations on somebody else the mothers can then try touching their own limbs.

Sheila Kitzinger (1977) uses touch in a different way which has strong psychological overtones. She likes to work with a husband and wife team. The woman lies on her side and the man stimulates the sensory nerves of her back by tapping or clapping down the length of the long back muscles. He is then asked to keep his hand still over what would be a painful area in labour while the woman relaxes towards the feeling of warmth and comfort of her partner's hands. This may be a very effective method of conveying support and sympathy in labour.

Some teachers rely on verbal imagery to describe the required sensations of bodily ease; for example 'Imagine your leg is getting heavier, or warmer, or your body is spreading outwards or you are floating on water'—these suggestions usually being given in a very calm, soothing monotonous voice. In certain types of meditation relaxation is achieved not through any conscious control of muscles or joints but by concentration on breathing control and sometimes on a word or 'mantra'.

Other teachers prefer a more matter of fact approach. They may use Jacobsen's 'contrast' method of teaching relaxation. This relies on appreciating the sensations which arise from tense, contracted muscles and the change which occurs when these muscles are relaxed. A modified description of this method will be found on p. 97.

Laura Mitchell has given us the following description of her 'physiological relaxation', based on her interpretation of the physiological laws governing muscle action.

'The human brain acts like a computer. The output in muscular activity depends upon what information the brain is receiving either from outside or from within the body.

'If one wants to perform a movement like "Stand up" or "Run for a bus" for a purpose, the appropriate muscular tension is built up by nerves leading from the brain. The work is done and immediately the tension disappears. If, however, the incoming information to the brain is an emotional one of fear, pain, or apprehension as one often finds in the pregnant and labouring woman, the brain becomes part of this fear reflex. It sends out messages to muscles to prepare for fighting or running away.

'This stress reflex is very primitive, but the muscular tension being produced is obviously useless to deal with the situation. The tension builds up, and the patient can become exhausted.

'All bodily activities are performed in patterns of movement, either innate or learned. The pattern of muscular activity in stress can be clearly demonstrated. It is exact and affects the whole body. All muscles do not need to be relaxed, therefore, only those involved in making the stress pattern. Let us consider the arms. The shoulder girdles are raised, the upper arms are flexed and held close to the body, the elbows are flexed and the hands clenched—making a picture of the typical fighting position.

'To obtain relaxation from this pattern it is useless to say "relax" so one teaches the patient to apply for herself the law of reciprocal inhibition. Modern physiologists tell us this is "pre-programmed" in the nervous system. This means that if one group of muscles is contracted voluntarily, then the muscles which perform the opposite movement (the antagonists) must *relax*.

'Therefore, to change the stress position into one of ease, the patient is asked to lie on the floor, and is taught to give the following orders to her arms: "Pull the shoulders towards the feet." "Stop." "Feel the resulting position." "Open the elbows out and away from the sides." "Stop." "Feel the resulting position." "Make the fingers long and supported." "Stop." "Feel the resulting position."

'These orders have been carefully chosen so that the brain will work the muscles which will relax their tense opponents. One asks the patient to register the resulting position in *joints* because joints have so many nerve pathways leading to the brain registering position. Muscles have no pathways registering contraction.

'Appropriate orders are continued until the whole body pattern is changed. Messages flash up and down, removing tension and registering ease. Gradually a feeling of well-being spreads over the body so that parts of it may even discard their own tension (for example, eyes may close) before they are told to do so. In any case, if the whole technique is performed, total relaxation is the inevitable result.' (See Mitchell, 1977). Further details of this method will be found in Laura Mitchell's book *Simple Relaxation* and her tapes (see Appendix). If only joint positions can be registered by the brain it is not clear how sensations of contraction are transmitted in such areas as the scalp and pelvic floor. We find that at present neurophysiologists do not all agree on the exact pathways which are used.

In a long and detailed survey, both of his own recent experimental work and of the literature, McCloskey (1978) states that the classes of afferent fibres that are candidates for subserving kinesthetic sensibility are those from the skin, from muscles and tendons and from joint capsules and ligaments. After examining each of these in detail he concludes that 'the role of joint receptors in the senses of movement and position is doubtful. Anaesthetisation of joints impairs kinesthetic sensation only when accompanied by anaesthetisation of the overlying skin. Total replacement of joints with prostheses causes only minimal kinesthetic impairment.'

'The principal receptors subserving the senses of movement and position are intramuscular receptors, probably the primary and secondary endings of the muscle spindles. Of the evidence advanced over the past 25 years purporting to show that intramuscular receptors have no role in kinesthesia, none now stands unchallenged. Instead, positive evidence exists for a kinesthetic contribution from intramuscular receptors in both limb muscles and extraocular muscles. For joints in the fingers and toes the discharges of intramuscular receptors probably are facilitated centrally by discharges from regional cutaneous and possibly joint receptors.'

These differences in interpretation of the physiological findings may be the reason why different teachers seem to be equally successful with different methods of teaching relaxation. It seems that we should be aware of these and should vary our teaching to suit different patients.

We have not found bio-feedback machines, which register changes in skin resistance due to sweating, of much help in distinguishing between small amounts of muscular tension, though they are useful in noting degrees of emotional arousal.

It seems clear that if different teachers are equally successful with different methods, we should all be aware of these and should vary our teaching to suit different patients.

Organisation of material

As for a talk or discussion, the background material must be prepared; that is, the object and method of performance of each exercise or variation must be known. The former can be learned from lectures or a book, but there is only one way of learning the latter—to *do* it oneself and experience the required sensations. At first you need a sympathetic tutor to check your faults and then you practise at home in front of a mirror. Next comes the problem of how to teach the exercise to somebody else, and here the help of colleagues or family as a practice class is indispensable. They will be quite happy to show you that your instructions are not clear, or point out that they have been left holding their breath because you have forgotten to tell them to breathe out.

Presentation

Having explained the object of an exercise the easiest method to illustrate what you are talking about is to demonstrate it. The cunning ones manage to talk and demonstrate at the same time. If you are facing a class remember that they see a mirror image of the movement so that if you want them to raise their *right* arms you must say 'right arms, lift' while you raise your own *left* arm. Then the class is arranged in a starting position such that you can see everybody easily, perhaps all facing the same way or all facing in towards the centre of a circle, but if the women have a tendency to giggle they may be better facing *out* from the centre.

Give a clear word of command after a pause, for example, 'Breathe out and let—go', or 'palms of the hands together, elbows out, ready, —press'. One is not trying to be a drill sergeant but we have found that pregnant women, like others, appreciate a little organisation and like to know exactly what they are supposed to be doing. More important still, it is much easier to run one's eyes over the group to spot faults and correct them if they are all moving in the same direction at the same time. Breathing is the exception to the rule, and since everybody has her own respiratory rate, this is left to each individual. Inexperienced people have a tendency to hurry exercises, particularly of the pelvic floor; the solution to this is to do the exercise oneself and perhaps count for the class at the same time.

The voice

All the points relating to appearance, communication and voice production in the section on Talks are relevant here also. The voice is a particularly powerful instrument when teaching exercises since the class will respond to your tone. If you say 'relax' you must sound restful, and not irritable when somebody is not doing too well. In contrast, if you want more effort out of the class, put more effort into your voice; for example, in an antenatal class you might say 'pull your tummies in, let go', while in a postnatal class it would be 'pull in, hold it, HOLD IT and let go'.

Corrections

Move around and make contact with each member of the group. During the first one or two classes, corrections are best given in general terms; for example, 'Some of you are standing with your weight too far back on your heels', you demonstrate, exaggerating the fault, 'try to stand tall so that your bust line is in front of your tummies'. When you know the class better you will sense who can tolerate a little individual help and criticism, but beware of singling out one member of the group who is already different in her own eyes, maybe unmarried or coloured.

Working in pairs

We find that just as members of a group learn through talking to each other, they also learn through watching and touching each other, and are often less shy when experimenting with movements with a partner than in a row in front of a teacher. This form of practice seems to be particularly useful in relaxation training. Working with a different partner each week in a woman's class helps to integrate the class, and they support and encourage each other; it also seems to help to break down social and racial barriers. It is an obvious method of organising couples classes, though here it is important that both the man and the woman should take turns at being the pupil. Sheila Kitzinger (1977) describes a form of touch relaxation; she is particularly enthusiastic about the results when the partners can work together, both in class and in labour. She suggests a series of contractions of different muscle groups of the body which are commonly held tense under stress. In couples classes the partner then places his relaxed hands on the muscles to localise the area over which the woman should relax. Partners can become interested and involved by learning these manoeuvres, and they can use them to offer active support during pregnancy and prepare for their possible role in labour.

REINFORCEMENT

It is a good idea to spend a few minutes each week recapitulating the salient points from the previous class. One can preface one's remarks with 'Last week we talked about . . . , did it raise any questions after you got home, or does anything further arise that you would like to discuss?' Exercises always need a lot of repetition and can be made more interesting and useful if the basic movements are repeated in different starting positions.

A small number of the more intellectual members may take notes, but others will prefer to be offered duplicated notes or leaflets to which they can add their own reminders. A book list, or better still copies of suitable books, should be available for inspection but it is usually impossible to keep a class library owing to heavy losses. Notes and leaflets written by other teachers are never quite what one needs, and the experienced teacher will write her own.

Another potent source of reinforcement is from other people, maybe from an ex-class member, a distinguished visitor or a colleague who makes the same statements in slightly different words. 'Observers' can often contribute useful points from their own experiences.

Evaluation of learning

Evaluation of factual learning in groups of this kind is difficult since one is trying to get away from the teacher-pupil-school atmosphere and its standards. Occasional questions such as 'Does anyone remember what signs to look out for when you are approaching the end of the first stage of labour?' or, 'Does anybody recall the points to remember when you are giving your baby his first feed?' wake the class up and encourage them to think. But persistent questioning may make the duller members of the group feel inferior.

The best idea of what has really been assimilated probably comes from questions and discussions, or interchanges between two women who are practising together in a situation in which they think they are out of earshot of the teacher.

The performance of exercises and relaxation, on the other hand, is easy to evaluate, as is the improvement among those who practise. During later labour rehearsals it is a good idea to present the class with a situation and to ask them to show how they would cope with it. For example, 'You are walking back from the toilet and have a contraction in the corridor, what will you do?' or 'You are alone and you suddenly want to push, how will you cope?'.

Role-playing

This is a fairly modern method of teaching, but as it is used quite frequently in schools and colleges will be familiar to many class members. We all, to some extent, adopt role-playing in our teaching techniques. Here are a few instances.

In our second stage practising, to make it as real as possible, we try to mimic the midwife's encouragement as she urges the woman to push harder and longer, so that we ourselves assume the role of midwife in the rehearsal, and talk of seeing the baby's head—'It's got dark hair', etc. We may attempt an imitation of the baby's first cry, as the birth contraction is completed. We may also give some idea of the sound the suction machine will make in the seconds after the baby is born.

It is also a form of role-playing when we demonstrate on women how their husbands can help them with massage and support in labour. It is even more so when we encourage them to work in pairs, with one acting the woman in labour, and the other her husband. Working with parents together, on 'Fathers' evenings', the wife assumes the role of herself in labour, and the husband rehearses his support techniques with her.

One of us has recently given a morning's class on antenatal teaching to male health visitors, and as part of the purpose was to teach them how to describe the husband's role, and how he could help in labour when working with expectant parents, a male volunteer became the woman in labour, while the teacher became the husband giving support and massage. Space was limited, so there was no question of the whole class lying down, but by rehearsing different adaptations of breathing and relaxing while sitting on chairs, and second-stage breath-holding with chin on chest, they all said they had a great deal more insight into what labour was really like.

Most of these illustrations would be used by a teacher without consideration that she was using role-playing techniques.

Deliberate role-playing is the setting up of small dramatic scenes to illustrate certain points for discussion. It could be physical, the teacher demonstrating the position of having, for instance, her legs placed in stirrups for a surgical induction, and encouraging the class to verbalise their feelings about the position. It could be a verbal interaction between two teachers to convey feelings; for example, a short dialogue in which one acted a tired wife at the end of a day with a crying infant, the other the husband, also tired, and the pattern of altercation which might ensue.

In *Teaching and Training* by H. R. Mills (1972), he notes that some advantages of role-playing are that interest is easily aroused and held, and that the teaching is both visual and aural and can sweeten a tired or 'browned off' class. He says that there are disadvantages in the time and effort required for production, and the dramatic or humorous effects may be exaggerated, unless great care is taken. Following this, in the next paragraph, he notes that role-playing is more suited to teaching *attitudes* than skills or knowledge. As our antenatal teaching is very much concerned with attitudes, perhaps role-playing has a part. If it is being done in the 'dramatic playlet' sense, the teachers using it must know each other and their own attitudes to various situations very well. They must decide whether to learn a set script, or to have a few guidelines on the topic to make a spontaneous performance. Above all, it must be well rehearsed, and then given first in front of critical colleagues, who will be honest in their assessment of acting ability and whether the reality of the situation has been conveyed. Without this, one could think oneself effective when in fact either overacting or appearing wooden and unrelaxed.

At the Third International Congress of Psychosomatic Medicine in Obstetrics and Gynaecology, in 1971, the first conference morning contained a beautiful piece of role-playing. An accomplished actress, speaking from a learned script, pretended to be a young woman waiting to see her doctor and learn whether or not she was pregnant. Her moving soliloquy contained the doubts, fears and hopes of most women in this situation, and gave many male obstetricians present more empathy and understanding.

We can see that a playlet of a health visitor talking with a new mother could be of value, if the 'health visitor' came over as warm and helpful, while the 'mother' was very inquisitive, and perhaps a little stupid, so that answers could be simple, all the class could follow, and many questions they may have thought of could be answered.

Other useful playlets could be:

1. The first visit to an antenatal clinic (this to be in a very early class before the women have had hospital experience).

2. A dialogue between a midwife and a mother coming to hospital in labour, the midwife reassuring but rather 'official', the mother rather hesitant, not remembering events of early labour too well.

3. A dialogue between a mother with 'postnatal blues' and another who has come through them and gives encouragement.

4. A dialogue between a breast-feeding and bottle-feeding mother in hospital.

5. A conversation between a 'husband' who has supported his wife in labour and watched his baby's birth, and another 'husband' who is ambivalent, and feels he might not be of use.

6. A discussion between a midwife from a 'high technology' hospital and a mother wanting 'active birth', to see if the two can come to a meeting-point acceptable to both.

We therefore think that role-playing, if used with confidence and care, has value, and should at least be considered as a teaching technique.

Teaching couples who do not know English

During Adult Education courses in 'English as a Second Language' it was found that new ethnic groups in the country have an urgent need to learn how the Health Service works, before they have assimilated enough English to understand anything written in ordinary booklets, pamphlets, notices, etc.

To give non-English speakers a knowledge of the Health services available, the BBC has published a book which is obtainable in twelve languages—Italian, Spanish, Portuguese, Greek, Turkish, Arabic, Bengali, Gujarati, Hindi, Punjabi, Urdu and Chinese. This is entitled *Your Right to Health* (Lo, 1982) and is at present available from Health Education Departments and local libraries, though the producers have suggested other outlets, such as shops in immigrant areas, places of worship, and self-help organisations. The BBC also suggest that hospitals, schools, health centres, GP's surgeries, and citizens' advice bureaux should have the books available.

It would be a great help to midwives, and to all who teach antenatal classes, to know that the persons they were advising had read the book and understood it, as they could then work with the knowledge that they had received the following information about childbirth:

GP services to confirm pregnancy and give antenatal care
Birth in hospital or home, consultants, GP or shared care
Routine antenatal care, clinics and classes. Nutrition
Benefits—free dental treatment and prescriptions. Maternity grant
Low-income—free milk and vitamins, fares, supplementary benefits

Working mothers—time off for clinics, maternity allowance and maternity pay.

The birth:

Admission into hospital. Labour. Fetal monitors. Birth positions. Pain relief. Speeding up labour. Forceps deliveries. Caesarian section.

After the birth:

Baby with the mother. Nurseries. Special care units. Breast and bottle feeding.

Roles of midwife and health visitor.

Registering the birth.

With the English and foreign versions together, an antenatal teacher and a non-English-speaking couple could use the texts, with added pictures and body-language, as effective teaching tools.

The pictures could be the Birth Atlas, Cow and Gate flip chart, or simple drawings or cut-outs from booklets, and the teacher could use her body, with a doll, to demonstrate progress in labour, positions, relaxation and breathing.

This type of teaching is probably only effective with one or at the most two couples together, so that their individual needs can be met.

If a woman can go to hospital, even without verbal communication, with a knowledge of what may happen, and her own pictures and diagrams to make herself understood, the one-to-one teaching can go on, with her midwife coaching her through contractions by example and imitation, and her partner helping her to make the staff aware of her needs as labour progresses.

This takes time, but creates a climate of confidence in an immigrant group, and a willingness of more couples to come to learn how to conform to some of our routines while still keeping to their own traditions and culture.

Teaching by pictures, and learning a rudimentary amount of English in the shortest possible time, is described in an article by Gill Thorn (1982) who worked with Vietnamese pregnant refugees.

REFERENCES

Abercrombie, M. L. J. (1970) *Aims and Technique of Group Teaching*, Teaching Methods No. 2. London: Society for Research into Higher Education.

Beard, R. (1970) *Teaching and Learning in Higher Education*. Harmondsworth: Penguin.

Kitzinger, S. (1977) *Education and Counselling for Childbirth*. London: Baillière Tindall.

Klein, J. (1961) *Working with Groups*. London: Hutchinson.

Lo, J. (1982) *Your Right to Health* (English version: *Their Right to Health*).
  London: BBC Publications.
McCloskey, D. (1978) Kinesthetic sensibility. *Physiological Reviews*, **58**, 4.
Madders, J. (1980) *Stress and Relaxation*. London: Martin Dunitz.
Mills, H. R. (1972) *Teaching and Training*, 2nd edition. London: Macmillan.
Mitchell, L. (1977) *Simple Relaxation*. London: Murray.
Thorn, G. (1982) Teaching the boat people. *New Generation*. London: National
  Childbirth Trust.
Wagstaff, G. (1982) A small dose of commonsense. Communication & persuasion in
  physiotherapy. *Physiotherapy*, **68**, 10.

FOR FURTHER READING

Argyle, M. (1967) *The Psychology of Interpersonal Behaviour*. Harmondsworth:
  Penguin.
Auerbach, A. (1967) *Parents Learn Through Group Discussion*. New York: Wiley.
Bessell, R. (1971) *Interviewing and Counselling*. London: Batsford.
Dunkin, E. (ed.) (1981) *Psychology for Physiotherapists*, Ch. 3. London: Macmillan.
Hellier, M. (1971) *The Art of Saying a Few Words*. Macmillan Journals. Available
  from F. P. A. Book Centre, 29 Mortimer St., London W. 1.
Jacobsen, E. (1977) *You Must Relax*. London: Souvenir Press.
O'Connell, A. & Gardner, E. (1972) *Understanding the Scientific Bases of Human
  Movement*. Edinburgh: Churchill Livingstone.
Sydney, E. & Brown, M. (1961) *The Skills of Interviewing*. London: Tavistock
  Publications.

3

Audiovisual aids

In this television-ridden age we are accustomed to having every fact illustrated, every emotion pictured, so the parents who come to our classes expect visual material of a high standard. The intellectual ones are used to learning from books and lectures, others may never listen to talks or read anything but picture papers and comic strips. In either case, far more people have visual rather than auditory memories—as Confucius said, one picture is worth a thousand words.

Pictures and diagrams help to clarify physiological processes, to emphasise points of importance, and to show situations outside the confines of the classroom. The hygiene of pregnancy is much more vivid against a background of shopping, cooking and gardening; the care of a new baby comes to life when a real baby is introduced to the class, or failing that an attractive film sequence. With the exception of the sounds accompanying a delivery, particularly the baby's first cry, pictures have a much higher emotive effect than sounds, hence their dangers but also their value in aiding memory and triggering off discussion.

Sources of material

Cost, availability and ease of transport are all important factors in determining what can be used. County health education officers and medical school librarians often have stores of material and equipment unthought-of by those who work on the periphery. This wealth of material and expertise should be known and used. It is possible to borrow film projectors, overhead projectors and even video equipment in many departments, together with the latest films and slides, and to get the latest leaflets and booklets for distribution to our classes. Since the new Health Districts were formed in 1982, hospital and community have been drawing even closer to each other and sharing facilities. This means that a midwife, based in hospital, can use her community Health Education Department as a resource centre, and a health visitor or physiotherapist in the community can have access to hospital libraries, and also to lectures by visiting specialists in the hospital, to keep up-to-date in her chosen field. Many drug and baby-food manufacturers will lend their films free of charge, and some will even supply a projectionist. Most slide and filmstrip producers will send their wares on approval. Technical colleges, schools and camera clubs are sources of projectors and record players of various kinds. Many shops will loan baby equipment for demonstration purposes.

The National Childbirth Trust publishes a *Teaching Aids Catalogue* which was being revised at the time we went to press. Some additional aids have therefore been inserted at the end of this chapter, together with a list of useful addresses.

Choosing audiovisual aids

As with all other facets of this work, we are faced with groups of people who may have widely different cultural backgrounds and therefore may be affected in very different ways by the material presented to them. One girl may find a picture of an embryo a fascinating bit of scientific information, another will dislike it intensely because it conflicts with her own image of her growing baby.

One golden rule seems to be that any picture or model of a baby must be attractive. Dolls, if used, must be as life-like as possible and must always be handled with the loving care one would give to a real baby. Secondly, the parents should be able to identify with those in the pictures. This means that visual material requires frequent renewal as clothes and hair styles change. A few notable attempts, such as in the filmstrip 'Your First Baby' and the film 'Preparing for Sarah' have been made to picture mothers and babies of different races, but we are woefully short of material for Afro-Asians. Colour is highly evocative, some people find green placentas (as shown in one teaching aid) unattractive, and blood always looks peculiarly 'bloody' on colour slides. Humorous drawings can make a point, but a woman with, for example, poor posture, needs to be so grossly caricatured that no member of the audience would accept that it could be her.

Commercially produced teaching aids are expensive and are never exactly what one wants, so many of us are driven to produce our own. Simple movements of the hands can be used to illustrate

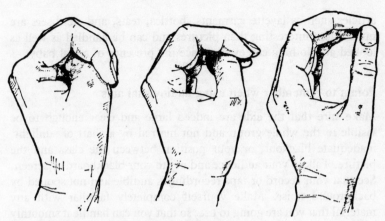

Fig. 1 Use of hand to show progressive dilatation.

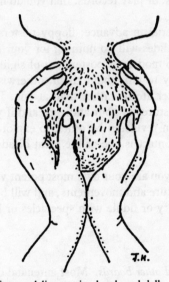

Fig. 2 Simulation of forceps delivery using hands and doll.

dilatation of the cervix (Fig. 1), and spontaneous and instrumental delivery (Fig. 2). Diagrams that grow either by altering lines on a blackboard or gradually building up a flannelgraph picture are easier to understand than a completed drawing. Mothers often find it easier to remember a diagram that they have themselves completed; for example, they can be given a series of outline contraction waves and asked to fill in the kinds of breathing they have learned. Actual articles such as layette garments, bottles, teats, and sterilisers are much more interesting than pictures and can be handled as well as looked at. Nothing can ever replace the presence of a real baby.

Points to remember when using audiovisual aids

Make sure that the aids are indeed large and clear enough to be visible to the whole group and not marred by a shaft of sunlight, inadequate blackout, or your position between the class and the picture. Talk to your audience and not to your blackboard or screen. See that your record or tape recording is audible and not spoiled by background noise. Make yourself completely familiar with any material that you are going to use, so that you can handle it smoothly and interestingly, prepare your commentary to make the most of its salient points and think out suitable leads towards discussion. *Never* show films or slides, or play records, that you do not know, however well recommended.

Prepare all material in advance; floppy posters, missing dusters and upside-down slides will do nothing for your image or anybody else's. But do keep models or posters out of sight of your audience until you are ready to talk about them, otherwise all eyes will be staring at the model uterus rather than at you. Finally, watch the expressions and gestures of your audience and if you note a look of puzzlement or even revulsion be quick to explore the reason. The lack of audience contact is one of the great disadvantages of sound film.

Remember that you are your own most potent visual aid, the class will copy your posture and movements, and will be distracted if you wear flashy jewellery or fiddle with spectacles or hair.

USEFUL AIDS

Chalk boards and other boards. Most antenatal clinics and centres have a blackboard and coloured chalks available; if not, a smooth piece of wood with a double coating of blackboard paint makes an acceptable substitute. Some health centres will have Magiboards— smooth white boards which make excellent surfaces for drawing with water-soluble pentels. Failing these, a piece of hardboard with white Fablon from Woolworths makes a good surface for drawing with water-soluble pentels. The drawings can be removed with a damp cloth.

Overhead projectors can be used as a more sophisticated form of blackboard. Words and drawings are outlined on a roller with water-soluble colours and projected on to a wall screen; blackout is not necessary. Writing in the normal size and hand position is easier for the teacher and pentels are much less messy than chalk. Drawings can also be prepared in advance.

Episcopes are similar to overhead projectors but cheaper; they cannot be used for free-hand drawing but will reproduce previously prepared material, leaflets, cut-outs or pages from a book. The teacher must be careful to arrange the sequence of pictures well ahead, especially if she is going to use several from one book.

Flannelgraphs have the advantage that the teacher does not need to pay attention to drawing, thereby turning her back on the audience, but can face the group all the time. A simple, colourful flannelgraph of human reproduction is available from the International Planned Parenthood Federation. Personal flannelgraphs, illustrating, for instance, the food which makes up a good diet, are easily made by cutting out suitable pictures, backing them with flannel or felt and pressing them on to a felt-covered board. Alternatively 'plasti-graphs' of transparent coloured plastic cut-outs will adhere to a plastic-covered board.

Charts, posters and pictures. Some of these are already mounted to stand easily on a table, such as the Cow & Gate Mothercraft Teaching Aid, or the SMA breast and bottle feeding charts. These both have strong metal spirals for their flip-over pictures. The Maternity Center Birth Atlas is in book form, but again is designed to stand well, and the pages can be seen clearly by a group of up to a dozen people. Other posters and pictures are better mounted on hardboard and rested on an easel. If they need to be rolled and transported from place to place, they can be protected instead by a plastic film such as Takibak.

Slides, filmstrip and *film* all require more sophisticated apparatus but they do have an element of drama absent from other pictorial forms. Unless daylight screens are used, a good blackout is essential. Slides are the most adaptable since their order and the commentary that goes with them is infinitely variable. A sensible assistant to act as projectionist is helpful and she should be provided with the slides, either marked with a spot in the bottom right-hand corner or better still with reversed slides arranged in order in a rack. If available, an automatic projector which can be loaded in advance (the Carousel takes 80 slides) and focused at a distance, thus allowing the teacher to watch her audience, is very useful.

Filmstrips are more easily transportable than slides and they cannot get out of order but only the commentary can be varied. Flipping over a frame is not a good idea since the audience is always suspicious that it is something nasty. To show filmstrips it is necessary to obtain a non-automatic slide projector with a filmstrip adapter. The strip needs to be inserted upside down and backwards. All film strips have an accompanying booklet, and some have taped commentaries which can be purchased separately.

Film. Television has made all of us much more sophisticated in our expectations. Recently, all channels have shown some aspects of pregnancy and birth. Because of the amount of money available for television projects, these have been attractive, well made and completely up-to-date. Films, which can be hired or bought by Health Departments or parenthood organisations, inevitably suffer by comparison, because they are used for too long and quickly become 'old-fashioned'. It may be argued that parents need to be prepared, in a class situation, with the reality of birth before their eyes, but it is rare to find a couple now who have not seen some of the media presentations of different aspects of labour. If they have *not* seen birth on television, it may be because they have wished to avoid it—so why should we thrust a film in front of them in a situation where it is difficult to escape? It is also very different to watch a film, in glorious colour, than to be holding hands together in labour and going through the experience. Coping with the latter is often much easier, with the father who imagined he would feel squeamish becoming completely involved in helping his wife.

The tendency, now, for those who think film can be valuable as a teaching tool, is to use 'trigger' films—short, sometimes controversial portrayals of situations which are designed to promote discussion. Examples of some of these will be found in the Appendix.

However, in this age of small, nuclear families, many prospective parents will have very little experience of babies, or any knowledge of what babies can do and perceive from birth, and how they react to situations. Films are now being made showing the responses and abilities of the newborn, and we feel that these are valuable to all those parents who have had little opportunity of observing and handling young babies. A film such as *The Amazing Newborn* (see Appendix) encourages the new parent to be sensitive to the baby as a person from the first days of life.

Films are, of course, expensive and fragile, and should always be shown and rewound by a skilled projectionist using familiar equipment.

Any film used in class must be known by the teacher, and appropriate to fill a gap in a teaching schedule. It is well to remember that parents give their whole attention to the expression and actions of the filmed parents—they are hardly conscious of the delivery techniques, which may be the first consideration of the professionals.

Film loops are a very easy way of showing short film sequences to small audiences. They need no threading up or rewinding since they are permanently mounted inside a cassette, but they do need special projectors some of which have a small translucent screen like a television set. They are also available with some of the 'Camera Talks' film strips to illustrate special sequences involving movement.

Records are now available for antenatal instruction. Some attempt, with the help of diagrams, to replace instruction from a teacher for those who are unable to attend classes. Others use a teacher's voice to encourage practice of relaxation and breathing techniques. These may be useful if the previous instruction has been along the same lines, but otherwise would be muddling. Records or tape recordings of an actual birth, which can convey in sound the atmosphere of a controlled and happy delivery and the excitement of the baby's first cry, make fascinating listening. Several cassettes and tapes are now available, dealing with relaxation and actual labour experiences. (See list at the end of this chapter.) An experienced teacher would never, however, play a cassette without discussion, and, of course, would be very familiar with the material herself. They can be used to reassure parents who picture labour as 'one long scream' and to help them to think themselves into the roles of the recorded parents and discuss how they would react in similar circumstances.

Models are helpful when something such as a pelvis has to be looked at in two dimensions, but they are expensive. A bony or plastic pelvis needs to be presented to the group in differing positions so that they can appreciate its make-up. It can then be held against the demonstrator's body and the watchers can feel the bony points on their own bodies. It is now possible to buy an accurate but very expensive model of the pelvic floor muscles; a good substitute, however, can be made of the fabric of an old girdle pierced by the three openings and marked by the guarding sphincters. This can be attached to the model and removed without a mark with Blu-tack, a plasticine-like adhesive obtainable from W. H. Smith and Sons. A useful mock-up of a pelvis can be made either from a plastic bowl with a hole cut in it or from two layers of stiff brown paper moulded on to and cut out from a model pelvis. This can look surprisingly realistic and the latter will pack flat if it needs to be transported.

A modification of the pelvis and floor model was first suggested by Sheila Kitzinger and is widely used by members of the National Childbirth Trust. She originally used a shoe box as the 'pelvis', cut an oval hole in the bottom of the box, and covered both the inside and outside with a thin layer of plastic foam from Woolworths. The 'baby' can be delivered through a slit in the foam. A more realistic model which is well worth the extra trouble required to make it can be produced as follows. Buy a plastic mixing bowl about eight inches in diameter and cut a circular hole in its base about two inches in diameter larger than the largest measurement of your doll's head. This is a tedious operation but can be done with a fretsaw or a hot knife. Stick a ring of thin plastic foam over the inside of the bowl so that it overlaps the rim of the opening by about half an inch. On the outside of the bowl stick a circle of plastic foam with a slit long enough to allow the doll's head to pass through. Araldite will stick the foam to the plastic, and the two foam layers together, without difficulty. The double layer hides the edge of the opening and the single layer in the centre bulges most effectively like a perineum. With a little experimentation to get the measurements right, it will open realistically to allow the doll to be delivered through it (Fig. 3).

Knitted uterus. A cheap and effective model uterus can be made from a pear-shaped knitted bag. The pattern was designed by a member of the staff of the New York Maternity Center and is now obtainable in this country through the Association of Physiotherapists in Obstetrics and Gynaecology (for the address see the end of the chapter). We find that the model is more realistic if filled with a balloon rather than being stuffed with old stockings as in the pattern, and that a double row of shirring elastic easily controls the opening to the 'external os' so that the ball or doll's head cannot fall out. It is useful for showing the effacement and dilatation of the cervix achieved by 'contractions', by squeezing the balloon. A simpler but less effective model can be made with the top of a sock, or the polo neck of a child's jersey.

Models of fetal development. These beautiful plastic models show the fetus *in utero* at different stages of pregnancy, and at full term. The pregnancy models (eight in all) show pregnancy from one month to eight months, with the baby in different positions—vertex, transverse, breech—and a twin pregnancy. In the later-stage models, the fetus is removable. The full-term fetus is also removable.

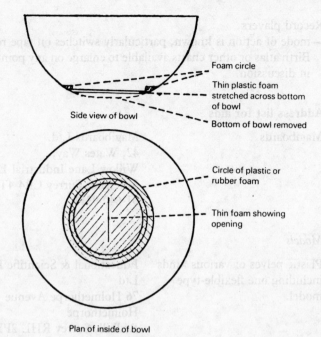

Foam circle

Thin plastic foam stretched across bottom of bowl

Side view of bowl

Bottom of bowl removed

Circle of plastic or rubber foam

Thin foam showing opening

Plan of inside of bowl

Fig. 3 Improvised pelvis using a plastic bowl.

Check list

Make sure that you have the following:

A quiet room arranged so that all can see and hear, well aired before blackout is done.

Blackboard

—coloured chalks

—duster

Models and charts

—table or easel to put them on

—spare balloon for knitted uterus

Slides, film, etc.

—you or your assistant must know how the projector works

—plug is correct for the socket, with plenty of flex for easy positioning

—spare bulb for lamp

—slides are marked with spot in bottom right-hand corner and in rack ready for loading

—position of light switches is known

—spotlight or torch to read notes if needed.

Record players
—mode of action is known, particularly switches on tape recorder.
Birth atlas or other charts available to enlarge on any points raised
in discussion.

Address list for aids

Magiboards	Magiboards Ltd. 42, Wates Way, Willow Lane Industrial Estate Mitcham, Surrey CR4 4TA. 01-640-9311.

Models

Plastic pelves of various kinds including one flexible-type model.	Educational & Scientific Plastics Ltd 76 Holmethorpe Avenue Holmethorpe Redhill, Surrey RHL 2PF Redhill 6278718
Pelvic floor for plastic pelvis	Ditto
Plastic or bony pelvis with ligaments also available from	Gerrard Biological Centre Gerrard House Worthing·Road, East Preston West Sussex BN16 1A5 090 62 72071
Models of fetal development mentioned in text Pregnancy set Full term model	Adam Rouilly Crown Quay Lane Sittingbourne, Kent ME 10 3 J G 0795 71378

Dolls

Fetal dolls with and without a placenta are available from	T. Gerrard & Co Adam Rouilly
Dolls for baby care	Vickers Ltd

Anne Baby

Priestly Road
Basingstoke, Hampshire

Other dolls of various ages
and weights from

Adam Rouilly
T. Gerrard & Co

Cheap floppy dolls which will
go through a pelvis are very
difficult to find. Gerrard's
make one which is described
as 'a flexible foam rubber
replica' of a new born baby
and appears to be more
attractive than most fetal
dolls. However, many good
toy shops now have flexible-
attractive baby dolls, which
can be used in a teacher's
hands, or against her body to
demonstrate positions and
manoeuvres.

T. Gerrard & Co

Rag doll patterns and kits
with white or black faces.

Needlework and Embroidery
Shops

Charts

Birth Atlas (Dickinson
Belskie) published by
Maternity Center, New York

H. K. Lewis & Co Ltd (and
N.C.T. headquarters)
136 Gower Street
London W.C.1
01 387 4282

A Baby is Born, a small birth
atlas in book form which
includes a breech birth

Compendium Bookshop.
234, Camden High Street,
London, N.W.1.
01-485-8944.

A New Life, 35 charts
illustrating all aspects of
childbirth and mothercraft.
This has recently been

Film Librarian
Cow & Gate Ltd
BA 14 8YX
Trowbridge, Wilts

changed and enlarged, to include fathers, an epidural, and more aftercare.

Stand for same

Relations of Growing Fetus to Other Organs. 4 black and white paper charts 17 × 28 in showing how mother's body adapts to growing baby

Many charts of male and female reproduction, some printed on paper, some on linen with rollers.

Charts of the normal birth process are produced by both Rouilly and Gerrard. The former have two charts No. 1 and 2, *Anatomical Changes in the Pelvic Contents*, which could be used by a new teacher unable as yet to afford an atlas. They also make two good charts of the male and female sex organs with transparent overlays, showing the development of the sperm, and the changes in the ovum and uterus during the menstrual cycle.

S.M.A. Breast and bottle feeding charts.

02214 68381.

Schuchardt Charts by Maternity Center
National Childbirth Trust
9 Queensborough Terrace
London W.2
01 229 9319

T. Gerrard & Co

Adam Rouilly

Wyeth Parentcraft, Wyeth Laboratories, Huntercombe Lane South, Taplow, Maidenhead.

The 'Sougy' obstetric series are intended for professional use but those charts showing breech (two) and twin presentations might be useful.

Adam Rouilly

Flannelgraphs

Flannelgraph of human reproduction including birth.

Purchasing & Distribution Officer
AV Production Services
International Planned Parenthood Federation
18–20, Lower Regent Street, London. SW 1Y 4PW.

Nutrition flannelgraph—basic nutrition presented in a colourful and interesting way.

Heinz Service for Schools
Hayes Park
Hayes, Middlesex

Shopping for Food

Records

The Expectant Mother, Long playing record or tape. *The Expectant Father*. Long playing record or tape. Betty Parsons.

Micronetro Ltd
PO Box 475
London NW10

Cassettes

Journey Thro' Birth
Shelia Kitzinger
Two cassettes

The Manor House,
Standlake,
Witney,
Oxon.
086 731 266.

Relax
Jane Madders
One cassette

Relaxation for Living,
29, Burwood Park Road,
Walton-on-Thames,
Surrey.
09322 27826.

Relief of Stress and *Teaching Antenatal Mothers*
Laura Mitchell
Two cassettes

Miss L. Mitchell, MCSP, Dipl TP
8 Gainsborough Gardens
London NW3
01–435 9337

Stress Management in Early Parenthood and *Nerves*
Lorraine Vines
Two cassettes

Twentieth Century Library of Recorded Education Ltd
Aqua House,
24, Old Steine,
Brighton.
Sussex.

Other titles on application for list.

4

Equipment and planning of classes

Most teachers have to make the best of the space allotted to them for classes, and in many cases it is far from satisfactory, but a number of new clinics and maternity units are now being built, so it may be useful to consider an ideal set-up. The location chosen should be within easy reach of public transport and have some car parking facilities of its own. There is, of course, no reason why the unit need be used exclusively for parentcraft classes but at the time that these are being held the group should have available to it a classroom, cloakrooms, a pantry for making tea or coffee, a small private office and, if two classes are to follow each other without a break, a waiting room. If fathers' or film evenings combining several classes are envisaged, then a room large enough to hold the expected number of couples will be needed.

ACCOMMODATION

The classroom should be large enough to accommodate the mothers comfortably, and have enough space to allow them to lie down while the teacher moves around. A very large room, however, has a cold, impersonal atmosphere—we would suggest a minimum free floor area for each woman of 2 m by 1 m (6 ft by 3 ft 6 in.) A rectangular room is easiest for teaching exercises.

There will be many occasions when the women in class will need to be lying down together—while teaching relaxation and antenatal and postnatal exercises, for instance. However, due to the diversity of equipment found in hospital today, and the different positions suggested in labour, at least two armchairs and several straight-backed chairs should be in the room. A table of convenient height, a couple of small stools, and perhaps even a bucket (see p. 169) should be available, with, of course, lots of pillows.

The room should be able to provide space for the women to move around, to change places with each other, and to find positions where they feel comfortable. They may like to remain sitting on their mattresses with their backs supported by pillows against the wall for talks and discussions or to sit in a half circle of chairs.

The room needs to be warm and well ventilated but free from floor draughts. Old fashioned sausage-shaped bags filled with sand are very useful for mitigating draughts under doors. Diffuse lighting is much more restful to the eyes than direct overhead lighting when one is lying on one's back but it must be strong enough to make pictures or diagrams clearly visible. A very sunny room may need curtains or blinds so that a shaft of light does not dazzle any member of the group. Blankets may be used as practice mats but rubber or plastic foam mattresses are much more comfortable, and these should have removable covers of some gaily coloured washable fabric. Loops at each end of the covers greatly facilitate handling. Plastic foam wedges sloping from a height of 20 cm to 5 cm (8 in to 2 in) on a 310 sq cm (48 in sq) base make excellent head and shoulder supports. Cylindrical bolsters may be used for flexed knees, but the mothers should not be encouraged to practise lying completely flat on their backs except for short periods. Pillows comfortably placed on the bolsters can give a half-side lying position where the uterus is partially supported. These bolsters may be filled with foam chips or be made of inflatable plastic bags similar to the buoyancy bags in a sailing dinghy. The latter are easy to store flat but if they have to be inflated frequently, a small hand or foot pump is a great advantage. If wedges and bolsters are not available, each mother will need at least three pillows, two for the head, one of which can be quite small (about 45 cm by 30 cm, or 18 in by 12 in) and one for the knees. Plastic pillow cases used in some clinics are hygienic but slippery and cold to the touch. Nylon seersucker or brushed nylon pillow cases are hard wearing and easy to launder. A few extra pillows will be needed to make somebody who has backache comfortable. Storage of mattresses and pillows can be quite a problem in a busy hall or clinic; the former should be kept flat, piled on a low broad shelf or hung from pegs against a wall. Further information about this equipment will be found at the end of the chapter.

If slides or films are to be used in this room, sockets for projectors and an adequate blackout are required. Most important of all, the room should be light and clean and have a welcoming air. Much can be done to improve an old one with bright posters or pictures of babies of different nationalities round the walls.

An office or small additional room is of tremendous value if the teacher wishes to have a private talk with a mother or couple and can be used as a rest room if somebody is feeling unwell. At least three comfortable chairs are needed and a desk for note-taking and records.

Cloakrooms. Adequate lavatory and washing space is a necessity wherever pregnant women are gathered together. Paper towels, with plenty of space for their disposal, and paper cups for drinking water are needed. Another lavatory at not too great a distance, which can be used by fathers, is greatly appreciated.

Equipment. Light but comfortable stacking chairs, as well as the straight-backed chairs already mentioned, are needed, so that enough seating can be provided for talks, especially when all the women's partners are present. One or two tables are invaluable for the display of leaflets and the accommodation of records and teaching aids. A blackboard fixed to the wall with a good supply of coloured chalks and an eraser is important, in addition to the other teaching aids which the teacher will buy or make. Cupboards with safe locks are needed for the storage of all equipment.

PLANNING THE COURSE

Getting a class together

Except during population fluctuations, good, established classes are rarely short of applicants, their worth is handed on from mother to mother but new courses may need hard background work and take time to build up. This is especially true if we are trying to interest foreigners, to whom the idea of preparation for childbirth may be new, or people who have recently moved into the area. The task is more difficult if we are also trying to prove the worth of such classes to sceptical maternity staff in the district. Consultant obstetricians, members of labour ward teams, GPs at booking clinics and sisters in antenatal departments can be approached in a number of ways, but preferably by the teacher in person. She will need to make her own opportunities for a preliminary approach to any of these people, possibly even seek their opinion of this book, but if she goes to a definite interview she must be well prepared to state her own aims clearly and offer a sample course programme for discussion. Physiotherapists are bound by their ethical bye-laws to accept patients only from a doctor but it is a great help if the doctor in charge of the patient's antenatal care is enthusiastic about the classes rather than merely permissive.

The National Childbirth Trust keeps a list of its own teachers and will refer an enquirer to the nearest class in her area or to similar organisations abroad. Staff in the units from whence it is hoped to draw patients should have clear and up-to-date information about the locale, days, times, starting dates, and booking arrangements of the courses and may be persuaded to put up a notice about these. Unfortunately many pregnant women, like railway travellers, do not read notices, and a few minutes spent by a staff member explaining the classes and how they can help is worth half a dozen posters. Names and addresses and expected dates of delivery of interested mothers should be noted so that a personal invitation to attend the first class of a certain course can be sent out. Alternatively, if mothers are coming from a single clinic they can be given a note confirming a date and time when they should come.

Six to 10 mothers seem to be the optimum number, as above 10 it is difficult to get to know the members of the group. Discussions are less interesting with less than six, although this will largely depend on the ability of the teacher and size of the room. Interpersonal relations become particularly important in these small groups.

Time and duration of classes

When planning the day and time of the classes, various points should be considered. In rural areas, or others where mothers must make a long journey, it may be helpful to hold the class on the same day as the antenatal visit. On the other hand, this may mean a lot of hanging about for some members of the group, and, if others require any special examination, they may miss the class. Such things as infrequent buses and cheap day fares should certainly be taken into account.

Daytime classes are desirable for both staff and primigravidae towards the end of pregnancy, but the latter may appreciate one or two evening classes earlier on and a fathers' class later. If both parents are invited to all the classes these will necessarily be in the evening. Multigravidae with children under school age naturally find daytime classes difficult; a friendly neighbour or a clinic crèche can solve the difficulty, but sometimes the only time these women will really either relax or concentrate is when the other children are at home 'with dad'.

We believe that the maximum duration of a class should be about two hours, and this should include refreshments, several changes of activity and possibly a change of teacher. After a two-hour session there should be at least half an hour's break before any one teacher is expected to begin another class, partly that she may recover her energy, and partly that several mothers may wait for the end of the class to ask privately about some point that has been worrying them. The tea break should be used as a time when the women can talk freely among themselves and make friends, but the teacher should be unobtrusively available and may indeed find herself making tea assisted by somebody who has a problem she wants to talk about.

Decisions as to what stage of pregnancy the women should start and finish the course offer a number of problems. There is little point in discussing diet, posture and the layette in the third trimester; on the other hand, preparations for labour and baby care are forgotten if learned too early. One would like to keep in touch with as many of the group as possible up to the time of delivery, but unless the syllabus is completed three to four weeks before the expected dates of delivery some will miss vital information due to pre-eclampsia or early induction. We have found that the best solution to these difficulties is to arrange one or two classes at about 16 weeks of pregnancy, one at least of which might be in the evening for couples. The rest of the course, including another evening for fathers, is then given between 28 and 36 weeks, and there is at least one refresher or continuation class open to women who have a month to go before their dates.

If classes are held only once a week and the course lasts for eight to 10 weeks, difficulties may arise in fitting in new people. It may be possible to start a second class in the week, thus giving a monthly intake, but if staff or numbers make this impracticable we believe that it is better to shorten the course while keeping it progressive rather than to take new people in continually. An exception may be made for allowing a woman to join the second class of a series but after that the group should be closed, except for those who have already done one course for their first baby and return for a 'refresher' of three to four classes.

Content of the course

The syllabus of each course will evolve gradually through trying to match the needs of the parents in the area, as these are revealed, to the staff and facilities available. Some suggestions are appended. Pregnant women need to go to the toilet frequently and are rarely comfortable for long in one position, so that several breaks and changes of position are desirable during any two-hour session, no matter what its content. Talks, discussions and exercises have been mentioned as the three methods of instruction commonly used in antenatal classes. If one teacher is responsible for the whole of the class the order in which these are used does not seem to matter much and may well vary either in the way a class develops and spontaneous discussions arise or according to which class is being taken. She may begin by talking or showing a filmstrip, encourage a discussion to develop, and finish with relevant exercises. Alternatively, she may begin by recapping the previous week's exercises while the late-comers get settled, then break off for a discussion, and pick up some particular point of interest that has arisen for a short talk. To finish she may go back to exercises again to highlight some point, for example the technique of pushing after a discussion on the second stage of labour. A refreshment break may thus be needed at different times. On the other hand, if two teachers are working consecutively with a group and their times and subjects must dovetail, much more definite structuring of each class is needed.

Classes where baby-care is completely divorced from the mother's care and reactions to childbirth do not on the whole seem desirable except perhaps for multigravidae, but if such a scheme exists there should be a frequent interchange of ideas between the teachers.

The first class is tremendously important and may well set the tone of the remainder of the course. Each mother, or if it is a combined evening class, each couple, should be welcomed by the teacher as guests rather than as patients, and information about them, if not already known, should be learned in a friendly and informal way. When the group has assembled, allowing a little time for latecomers in this first class, the teacher may introduce herself by name and tell the group why she is interested in antenatal education, perhaps including a remark about her own children if she has any. She may then ask the members of the group to introduce themselves, perhaps giving their full name, when and where they expect to have their babies, whether it is the first, and if not the ages of the others. If the group is a structured one, the teacher may then go on to tell the group its aims and briefly what is to be included in the course; alternatively, she may ask for their ideas on what aspects of child-birth they would like to have discussed. She will probably want to make the whole proceedings as informal as possible and to stress that questions will be welcome on any aspect, at any time, and it is hoped that the members of the group will share their experiences, ideas and reactions.

Records and follow-up

Essential information about each mother, such as her name, marital status, address, date and place of delivery, parity, and ages of other children, must obviously be recorded. It is useful to be able to refer to the medical notes, or at least to the mothers' continuation cards. Her occupation either before or during pregnancy is of interest, so is a brief history of other births and any salient points about her reactions to this one, for example, whether she feels fit and is happy about having the baby, how she plans to feed it, and whether she wishes her husband to be with her in labour. It may well be that these facts will emerge gradually during the course and there is a lot to be said for keeping a card for each mother in the class, instead of, or as well as, a simple register of attendance. The teacher can thus build up a picture of each mother or couple, including what questions they have raised, and their reactions to their problems, which will be of great interest to her and guide her in working with them.

Learning names is always a problem, but if a teacher is to gain real empathy with her group it is one which she must solve. Some teachers use first names, feeling that this is easier and adds to the informality of the class. We introduce ourselves by our christian and surnames and find that the class members quickly follow suit, they usually call each other by their first names, but we call them all by their surnames. An older teacher may well feel motherly towards a group of young women but we believe that, when young people are struggling to establish their identity in a new role, it is particularly important that helpers should recognise their new position by addressing them with appropriate dignity. All the women are called 'Mrs' unless they themselves make a point of their unmarried status. Some teachers like to ask their mothers to fill in name tags and to wear them, others resort to cryptic reminders on cards, such as 'tall dark secretary, usually wears red'. The leader who can quickly learn the names in her group by whatever means certainly has a tremendous advantage in showing her personal interest and care for each member.

The most exciting and educative follow-up to antenatal education is to be with a couple whom one has prepared in labour, at least occasionally, and to watch their first reactions to their baby. The work of any teacher who does not have this privilege tends to become uninspired and unrealistic. Next comes some form of personal contact after the baby is born, whether in the lying-in wards, in the home, or at the clinic where the mother's growing relationship with her baby, and any problems of adjustment that the couple may have, can be observed. Letters and telephone calls are second-best but still useful if the mothers are able to express themselves. They greatly enjoy a class reunion to which they take their babies about six to eight weeks after the last in the group has been delivered. If statistical results are required, these can only come from a carefully planned series of observations or reports derived from pretested questionnaires.

SUGGESTED OUTLINES FOR FOUR COURSES

Course 1

A very early class for primiparae.

One of us works in an area covered by nine family doctors. They find that, usually, a primipara attends for confirmation of pregnancy when her menstrual period is 2–3 weeks overdue. The local midwife and I talked to all the doctors, and they agreed to co-operate in asking all these women to bring their husbands to a discussion in the local clinic, as soon in pregnancy as possible.

Each doctor has a supply of letters, typed for us and signed by us, congratulating the parents on their pregnancy and inviting them both to an informal discussion evening. The letter states that we wish the pregnancy to be as healthy as possible and would like to give some advice about this, and that we are also available to answer any questions.

We meet twice a month, so as soon as a pregnancy is confirmed, the doctor checks the date of the next meeting, adds it to the letter, and encourages each couple to attend.

Response is good, and even if the group on one evening is fairly small, we still consider it worthwhile to be available at these set times. We do not know how many will arrive, but on average, five or six couples attend at each evening session.

In practice, we see the couples when the woman is between seven and ten weeks pregnant, just before she attends hospital for the first time.

Although we keep the group unstructured to some extent, to allow time for any queries or worries from the parents, we do give the following information at each evening's meeting:

Advice on diet, alcohol, cigarettes, drugs (with leaflets to take home).

Posture, exercise and relaxation (again with brief 'reminder' leaflets, prepared by ourselves).

Procedures at the first hospital attendance, and why.

Tests which will be done in pregnancy, and why.

We also give details of the different hospitals' methods, as appropriate, and of the hospital's classes and our own local classes, for later pregnancy, with dates, times and methods of booking. They take our telephone numbers for any further questions they may have in the coming weeks.

These evening groups have been running for less than a year, but we are now visiting the babies of the first sets of parents. So far, all reaction has been favourable—the parents have appreciated the time to talk in a relaxed atmosphere, and appear to have followed our advice on keeping healthy sensibly and readily. We are fortunate in being able to keep in contact with them during pregnancy, and they are pleased to see a midwife they know when they return home with their babies.

Course 2

A post-booking class in hospital for both parents.

The first class available may be the post-hospital booking class when the baby has matured to 12 to 16 weeks gestation. Many hospitals now offer an evening class for both parents at this time, often taken jointly by an antenatal sister and an obstetric physiotherapist; better still if an obstetrician, a dietician and a health visitor can be involved. The evening might well start with a welcome and a few words from one of the organisers about when the baby is expected, how the parents feel about it and any problems they may have encountered so far. It is well to remember that this may be the man's first contact with the hospital and his welcome may well colour his subsequent dealings with the staff.

We have found that slides are useful for catching the parents' interest during a fairly long evening and use a Camera Talks set called 'Pregnancy—A Challenging Experience'. These are 84 slides divided into two halves, Part I begins with the implantation of the ovum and goes on to picture the growth of the fetus up to full term. There are diagrammatic representations of the possible effects of the hormone changes on the mother's body, the routine care of the mother at antenatal visits is shown in pictures including weight checks and advice on diet and the use of ultra-sound. This part ends with a preview of later parentcraft classes and encouragement to attend.

Tea is served in the interval and we find it a good idea to have it on a central trolley so that parents can move about the room, talk to each other and to ourselves before settling down again.

The second half is concerned with self-help for the parents. It begins with six pictures illustrating emotional adjustments in mother and father designed to make them laugh a little and think a lot. Then come pictures of simple exercises the mother should do, suitable activities and the importance of good posture and lifting habits. Some positions for relaxation are shown and hints on relieving minor aches and pains such as cramp; and the series ends with some advice on the choice of shoes and bras.

At the end of the evening we make sure that mothers know when to come to begin the set of practical classes which we aim to finish approximately 2 weeks before their EDD. While clearing up the room we make sure that we are available to answer any questions that remain.

Course 3

Local Authority or private class, for mothers going to different units. Starting at 26–28 weeks of pregnancy.
1. Introductions
   Scope and purpose of the classes.
   Outline of reproductive system.
   Physical and emotional changes of early pregnancy.
   Practical: Correct posture and use of the body when standing, sitting, moving and carrying.
2. Further changes in pregnancy, including breast changes
   Discussion on feeding methods, breast preparation for those interested
   The importance of antenatal care, diet, sensible living habits
   Layette
   Practical: Recapitulation of posture, exercises for abdominal wall, pelvic floor and breasts: beginning general relaxation.
3. Signs of labour
   Contractions, what they do and may feel like, how to cope
   Practical: Relaxation with deep breathing in sitting, leaning and different lying positions; begin shallow breathing.

4. Later 1st stage of labour and signs of its end
   Coping with contractions as labour advances
   Drugs, analgesia including epidurals if available *Practical*: Relaxation with pelvic rocking for backache; various forms of massage; relaxation with deep to shallow breathing; broken rhythm breathing, tapping or counting if pushing reflex is established before full dilatation.
5. 2nd and 3rd stages of labour
   Appearance and early reactions to baby
   Practical: How to push or pant as requested.
6. Different patterns of labour including inductions
   Early development of baby
   Demonstration of holding baby in comfortable positions
   Beginning breast feeding
   Practical: Labour rehearsal.
7. The puerperium
   Hospital or home routine
   Demonstration of sterilising, making up feeds, etc. for bottle feeding.
8. Father's evening
   Film or slides and discussion on labour and puerperium
   How men can become involved and helpful
   Short talk or filmstrip on family planning.
9. Introduction of baby to class
   Bathing it
   Practical: Second labour rehearsal picturing some of the variations (e.g. an induction).
10. Taking the baby home, film, filmstrips and discussion to show its further development and routine
    Introducing baby to the family, changes in parents' lives
    Family planning (if not already done)
    Postnatal check
    Practical: Any points the class wishes to recheck, especially second stage of labour.

Course 4

Shorter course for mothers all booked at one hospital. Bathing, bottle-feeding, postnatal exercises, and family planning are not included since all are dealt with during hospital stay.

Starting at 16 weeks of pregnancy with an evening class for both parents.

1. Welcome—aims of the course
   Filmstrip such as 'Your First Baby', Part 1, with a good introduction.
   Discussion of physical and emotional changes of early pregnancy
   Diet and living habits to give baby a good start
   Choosing major articles of equipment (which will interest the men)
   Practical: Demonstration of good posture and working habits; simple relaxation and exercises sitting on chairs.
2. Recommencing at approximately 30 to 32 weeks
   Further changes of pregnancy including breast changes and preparation
   Discussion on feeding
   Signs of labour
   Layette on view for questions
   Practical: Recapitulation of exercises; general relaxation with deep breathing.
3. 1st stage of labour
   A shortened version of classes 3 and 4 in previous syllabus.
4. 2nd and 3rd stages of labour
   As for previous class 5.
   Different patterns of labour
   The newborn baby
   Practical: Labour rehearsal.
6. Second class for fathers
   Film or slides of labour and how fathers can help
   The puerperium and hospital routine
   Taking the baby home.
7. Hospital visit
   Talks with lying-in mothers, observation of babies and their feeds
   Practical: Second labour rehearsal.

Address list for equipment

Foam Camping Mattress	Blacks of Greenock Ltd
88 cm × 69 cm (74 in × 27 in)	3 Rathbone Place
56 cm × 188 cm (22 in × 74 in)	London W.1
	01–636 6645
	For local stockists write to
	Black & Edgington
	Ruxley Corner
	Sidcup, Kent

Nomeq make a number of different sized 'airex' foam gym mats which do not need covers, roll up and sponge clean

Nomeq
Melton Rd.
West Bridgford
Nottingham NG2 6HD
0602 23425

Relaxation pads
1.9 m × 0.9 m × 2.5 cm (6 ft 3 in × 3 ft × 1 in)
with fixed waterproof cover or loose cover with zip

Price Bros. Ltd
Wellington
Somerset

Wedges

74 cm × 38 cm × 20 cm (29 in × 15 in × 8 in) at back reducing to 1.3 cm (½ in) at front with covers

Ditto

Chiltern wedge

61 cm × 61 cm × 23 cm – 8 cm (24 in × 24 in × 9 in – 3 in)
61 cm × 61 cm × 41 cm – 0 cm (24 in × 24 in × 16 in – 0 in)
covers extra

Mrs. S. Redican
63, Aylward Gardens,
Chesham,
Bucks.
Chesham 785 802.
or through National Childbirth Trust

Labour Wedge for 2nd Stage
24 in × 24 in × 18 in
61 cm × 61 cm × 45 cm

As above.

Wedge covers

N.C.T. Headquarters.

Cushion

Posture Curve Cushion, about 46 cm (18 in) square, especially shaped to fit into and support lumbar curve, very comfortable for those with backache.

Sleep Centre
John Bell & Croydon
50 Wigmore Street
London W.1
01–935 5555

Bolster

Hexham Bolster. Inflatable air
cushion for underknee support.

Mrs J. Gibson
Linnel Hill
Hexham
Northumberland
Slaley 221

or through National
Childbirth Trust

5

Discussion of pregnancy

We cannot stress too often, or too forcibly, that a pregnant woman is vulnerable—that pregnancy, especially for the first time, is one of the major crises in a woman's life. In her first pregnancy she will change and grow emotionally, as well as physically. Some of the emotional growth will be through joy, anticipation and acceptance. There will be times when a woman will feel bubbly with happiness, perhaps as she feels the baby move, and times when she will go around dreamily in madonna-like serenity. She can imagine herself as the perfect mother, and discuss her pregnancy with delight. Thus she is accustoming herself to her new role. On the other hand, as teachers, we observe that pregnancy is at times difficult, and that some of the emotional growth may be achieved through apprehension and the overcoming of that fear.

All antenatal teachers, and in fact all who come in contact with pregnant women in a professional capacity, should remember that each woman will have times when she feels vulnerable, alone and afraid. She will also have feelings of ambivalence—even if the pregnancy has been eagerly desired and planned. Many women we meet, however, will have had to cope with an undesired pregnancy, perhaps a rushed marriage before which they will have experienced dismay, terror, a feeling of being trapped, parental disapproval and perhaps even a desire to abort. Some of the women will not be married, and may have little support from family and friends.

All, the fortunate and the much less fortunate, will have times when the realisation that their lives will never be the same again fills them with alarm. They may have to give up a challenging job and wonder whether caring for a baby will be a sufficiently satisfying occupation. There will also be the sudden, irrational fears—that they will fail as mothers, have an abnormal child, or even not survive pregnancy.

The pregnancy fills their thoughts, colours their whole attitude to daily life, and they become extraordinarily sensitive to words, brooding on the most casual remarks of obstetricians and giving them distorted meanings in many cases. One example of this was a woman from one of my classes whose obstetrician had said heartily and casually, 'That's a nice big baby you've got in there', and for weeks she worried about how it would get out, until her next hospital visit. This time she was examined by the registrar who, again casually, said, 'A nice compact baby here—not too big'. One would think she would be relieved, but in class she suddenly said she felt the baby must be abnormal, as it could not possibly be growing, recounting the two statements. Fortunately, the rest of the class had experienced similar light-hearted comments, and she was eventually reassured that both doctors were making casual conversation about a perfectly normal pregnancy

We can, as teachers, be aware of these stresses, and the excessive egocentricity of the pregnant woman. We can aim at truthful reassurance (always choosing words with exquisite care so that they are descriptive but not alarming) and a loving, caring attitude. We can give positive encouragement that she does her best, throughout pregnancy, to ensure her child's safety and wellbeing. By doing this, she is adopting a mature attitude and already 'being a mother', preparing for her coming role, and accepting that she is already responsible for another human being.

What does a woman want to know about pregnancy?

We suggest that the following questions are uppermost in most women's minds.

1. What is happening to my body?
2. How can I protect my baby and keep it healthy?
3. How can I adjust to this experience?
4. How can I remain as attractive and comfortable as possible in pregnancy and return to my normal figure afterwards?

In addition we need to tell her of the 'danger signs' which should be reported to her obstetrician or midwife.

METHODS OF PRESENTING THIS INFORMATION

We need to answer the factual questions, discuss the changes in attitudes, and teach the neuromuscular control which will help her to adjust her body to its changing weight and centre of gravity and to overcome stress by relaxation. Therefore, each class fits the preparation-for-childbirth triangle of a set talk with questions, a discussion period, and a period of practising neuromuscular control. We must also keep in mind the teaching triangle of teacher-class-subject, making sure that the teacher can present her material well, that the subject is relevant and important to the class, and given in such a way as to be interesting and attention-holding to that particular group. Because we do not intend, in class, to keep to a rigid schedule, it is possible that any topic could be discussed in any part of the course, depending on the needs of the members.

A flexible plan for information about pregnancy could be as follows. The first two points, 'What is happening to my body?' and 'How can I keep my baby healthy?', together with signs which need to be reported to obstetrician or midwife, could be covered by a set talk with questions, leaving plenty of time for clarification of points not understood. The third topic, 'How can I adjust to this experience?', falls naturally into a group discussion pattern. When covering the fourth topic, 'To remain attractive and comfortable and return to a normal figure afterwards', we would concentrate mainly on neuromuscular control.

Physical changes and health care (topics 1 and 2)

This would vary depending on the stage of pregnancy (see the syllabus examples) but could have the following headings.

Anatomy and physiology

This should be illustrated, wherever possible, by the Birth Atlas, Schuchardt charts, Cow & Gate pregnancy charts, blackboard diagrams, flannelgraphs, or filmstrips, and by the use of the teacher's own body and a model pelvis or even a large basin.

A brief and simple explanation of the size, position and shape of the reproductive organs, both non-pregnant and as pregnancy advances, with special reference to the protection the body gives and the adaptation of other organs throughout pregnancy.

The level of the fundus at different stages of gestation, and reasons for pressure symptoms, breathlessness, rib pains, bladder frequency.

Changes in hormone balance leading to the slowing of activity of unstriped muscles, perhaps causing constipation, haemorrhoids, varicose veins, indigestion. Ways in which these can be alleviated.

Breast changes. Muscle and joint changes, slackening of ligaments, with perhaps backache or pain in the symphysis pubis.

Changes in weight, balance, and centre of gravity.

The growth of the baby—size, weight, movements and heartbeats, and when able to survive independently.

The position of the pelvis and its relationship to the baby's head (together with terms used to denote the proximity of the head to the pelvis). The pelvic floor.

Professional antenatal care

This subject can be divided into the following topics:

The 'routine' questions and examinations, and their purposes.

Preventing abortion.

What is learnt in an early and a late pregnancy vaginal examination.

Blood pressure and urine tests and their importance in the early warning of pre-eclampsia.

Blood tests, and what they discover. Fetal monitoring. Alphafetoprotein measurements. Drugs in pregnancy.

The importance of checking the fetal heart rate, and the 'lie' and size of the baby. External version.

Ultrasonic echo sounding (ultrasound). Amniocentesis. Amnioscopy. Decompression.

Signs to report to the obstetrician or midwife, which ones are important and should be reported immediately, including any bleeding, losing liquor, headaches, disturbed vision, excess weight gain, loss of weight, oedema, regular strengthening contractions (with reassurance that early treatment will give the greatest possibility of continuing a normal pregnancy).

The mother's own care of herself and the unborn baby

This covers various aspects of health and hygiene:

Sensible eating, rest and exercise, with care that these are based on the educational, cultural, social and economic backgrounds of the group.

Shoes and clothes, including discussion of abdominal and breast support.

Nutrition in pregnancy.

Breast preparation.

Dental care and prevention of calcium deficiency.

Alcohol and smoking

As we are becoming more aware, from present research, of the vulnerability of the fetus, we must stress this to the mothers in our care. We have to do this, even if the knowledge is somewhat worrying, and causes deliberate sacrifice in changes in the mother's life-style, because the health of the child is indeed at risk.

There is no doubt now that nicotine passes to the baby and that he is, to some extent, poisoned by the cigarettes of a mother who is a heavy smoker or who is living in a cigarette-polluted atmosphere.

It has been found that, even if the mother smokes under 20 cigarettes a day, the baby will be smaller, and may have withdrawal symptoms after birth. In the major British survey of all children born in one week in 1958, it was found that the children of mothers who smoked were still statistically smaller at 7 years and 11 years of age, and did less well academically. A mother may need a lot of encouragement to stop, or cut down, smoking in early pregnancy, but the husband can help by stopping smoking with her (thus sharing in caring for the health of the baby) or certainly make it easier for her by not smoking at home.

Social drinking is now suspect, also. Recent research has proved that heavy drinking, or even the occasional party excesses, especially in the early weeks of pregnancy, can harm the normal growth of the fetus (Beattie, 1981).

It follows that we must, for safety, encourage women to use alcohol in moderation only, even on festive occasions. Fortunately, many women have a sudden dislike of alcohol, even before the pregnancy is confirmed. Perhaps this is one of the body's natural defence mechanisms

Naturally, if antenatal classes begin at the seventh month of pregnancy, we must get this information to the mother much earlier to be of any use at all. Many doctors discuss cigarettes, diet and alcohol as soon as pregnancy is confirmed. Other mothers depend on the midwife at the booking clinic, who talks to them about keeping healthy.

We have felt it worthwhile to have discussions in clinic with mothers, very early in pregnancy, where these points are stressed strongly (see pp. 18–19).

Recently, some family planning doctors have taught 'pre-conception healthy living', giving this information when women have attended, for instance, on stopping 'the pill' or on having their intrauterine device removed. This is the ideal time to think about preparing the body for childbirth.

Drugs in pregnancy

For a long time, the placenta was thought of as 'the placental barrier'. We know now that it is more like a complicated sieve, and that whatever a mother eats, drinks or smokes (including cannabis) will be passed, to some extent, through this sieve to the baby. We have stressed that no drugs whatsoever should be taken without the advice of the mother's doctor, but mothers have tended to think that any simple remedy, for headaches, indigestion, etc., which is bought in quantity over any chemists' counter, or picked up in the super-market, is safe. We know now that this belief is not entirely true. Studies have shown (Rosen *et al.*, 1978) that even the simple aspirin, taken at the end of pregnancy (for instance, for a cold, especially in the last week) may cause the baby to be anaemic when born, and much more likely to have jaundice (p. 192). So *all* medicines matter, and need a doctor's advice.

Any other topics arising from questions.

How can I adjust to this experience? (topic 3)

Changes in role and attitude can usually best be explored through group discussion, though this method of teaching can also be used for other parts of the syllabus. It requires a delicate sensitivity on the part of the teacher, to know when to let the group get side-tracked because this is benefiting the majority, or maybe even helping just one or two, and when, with a question or comment, she should bring the group back to the topics she has planned. The teacher, as group leader, should have an idea of the topics she intends to suggest, and may begin with a short talk or a filmstrip or film (for example, 'Your First Baby, Part 1, Pregnancy' or the first part of 'Preparing for Sarah'—see Ch. 3). She can then ask a few questions to encourage the participants, being prepared always to efface herself according to the group's needs, and to allow freedom in discussion.

Nutrition in pregnancy

Some mothers are wisely counselled by their doctors about their eating habits during pregnancy and lactation; others are just told that they are putting on too much weight or occasionally too little. Special problems, for example diabetes, will be referred to the dietitian for expert guidance, but every antenatal teacher should be familiar with some of the basic facts regarding nutrition during the childbirth cycle. Difficulties arise when one tries to find basic facts, since the experts disagree.

One of the major points at issue concerns the extent of a desirable weight gain during pregnancy. It is accepted that the additional weight of the uterus and its contents, also the breasts and blood is 8.1 kg (18 lb)–9 kg (20 lb), the argument begins over how much extra fat the mother should be allowed to lay down. Craddock (1978) says that a total of 9.7 kg (21.4 lb) is plenty of weight gain and that extra fat is unnecessary. He makes a case for giving dietary advice to any woman who gains more than 1.8 kg (4 lb) per month before the 20th week or 2.25 kg (5 lb) in any successive four weekly period thereafter. It is equally important that there should be a steady weight gain up to the 39th week. On the other hand, the authors of the Department of Health and Social Security's pamphlet *Eating for Health* (1978) says that the mother who by reducing her food intake, does not allow the normal increase in weight, may have a baby whose birth weight is less than it should be. 'Thus although a mother should not be allowed to become obese during pregnancy, she should expect an increase in weight of about 12.5 kg (27.5 lb). This allows for an increase of 4 kg (8.8 lb) of fat, this is enough energy to provide for the production of human milk for many weeks or months'. If overweight before pregnancy begins it may be advisable for a mother to gain less weight.

Perhaps we shall not go far wrong if we counsel our mothers to aim at a weight gain of 11.3 kg (25 lb) and bear in mind that those who are going to breast feed will lose weight more quickly. From the mother's point of view this amount will not usually cause stretch marks, backache due to poor posture or marked discomfort due to clumsiness.

The most dangerous period for weight gain due to fat is the second trimester after any early nausea is over, when a woman usually feels fit and hungry and is not yet so full of baby that she cannot eat a large meal. Even slim women sometimes gain a lot of weight at this time. It is widely accepted that a sudden weight gain in the third trimester is often due to fluid retention and may precede a rise in blood pressure and other symptoms of pre-eclampsia. These are more common in women who are either overweight before becoming pregnant or who have put on a lot of fat.

Some mothers in the classes will be very well aware of the constituents of a well balanced diet and will need to know only what their extra requirements are; for others, particularly the disadvantaged, this may be an opportunity to help them to plan their meals and to eat more wisely. In any case the teacher must be aware of religious taboos, cultural patterns and financial curbs among the group. For example it is useless to suggest that a Muslim woman should eat non-Halal meat, particularly pork, or a Hindu should use oily fish, and in some cases eggs, as extra protein. An excellent booklet called *Asians in Britain* will provide useful reference material on the dietary patterns in relation to their religious backgrounds of the various groups of Indians in this country.

When giving specific advice it should be remembered that it is mainly the requirements of proteins, minerals and vitamins which are increased during pregnancy. During the first half of pregnancy 10 per cent more protein both from animal and vegetable (legumes) sources should be taken. The changes in metabolism of the expectant mother cause the Vitamin A requirement to be increased and that of Vitamin C by approximately 100 per cent, necessitating the inclusion of extra dairy products and plenty of fresh fruit and vegetables. During the second half of pregnancy the rapid growth of the baby makes greater demands on the mother's nutritional reserves. The development of bones and teeth calls for extra supplies of calcium (over 100 per cent) and of Vitamin A and D. Milk, butter, or margarine, eggs and fatty fish should be taken. Additional Vitamins A, D and C are available without cost in tablet form to poor or large families under the welfare food scheme. Extra Vitamin D may be particularly necessary for Muslim women since they either go out heavily veiled or remain indoors away from any available sunlight.

The provision of extra iron in the mother's diet is also very important because the infant must store enough in its liver to last until it is weaned, though the Editorial in the *British Medical Journal* (1978) argues that iron supplements are not necessary for all women. Iron is more readily absorbed from foods such as egg yolk, meat, liver, dark green vegetables and wheat germ. However, tablets of iron and folic acid are usually well tolerated and their effect is increased if they are swallowed while eating a meat meal or with a Vitamin C-containing drink such as orange or grapefruit juice.

Suitable advice on diet for non-vegetarians is shown below.

Vegetarians are usually aware of the value of good eating, but should be reminded to keep up their protein intake by varieties of pulses, eggs, cheese and nuts.

Vegan mothers need special help, particularly in choosing foods that will give them an adequate supply of protein and Vitamins D and the B complex; these can if necessary be taken in tablet form. The Vegan Society, whose address is at the end of the chapter, will be glad to help with special diets for pregnant and nursing mothers.

We can point out to mothers who are keen to breast feed their babies that they can lay a good foundation for an adequate supply of milk by attention to their diet during pregnancy which will later need to be maintained during lactation. One pint of milk a day is said to lay the foundation for healthy teeth but Winter (1976) finds that there is at present no definite evidence that fluoride taken during pregnancy by mothers already on a good diet improves the condition of the baby's teeth. The situation is different after its birth.

Suitable advice on diet

Good eating habits are essential during and after pregnancy. This is to ensure that both you and your baby will be in the best of health. The quality of the food you eat is more important than the quantity. Regular meals of protein, fruit and vegetables are better than stodgy snacks and will help prevent an excessive increase in weight. You should not put on more than 9.5–13 kg (21–28 lb) during the whole of your pregnancy, and most of this should be in the later months.

Your menus should be based on the following foods:

Milk and cheese

These two products provide calcium which is essential for baby's bones and teeth. They also provide protein.

Increase your milk intake to 600 cc (1 pint) a day. Use it in milky drinks, puddings, sauces and on breakfast cereals. Yoghurt can also be used (1 carton = 1 glass milk). A piece of cheese three or four times a week is advisable.

Meat and other protein foods

Meat, fish, eggs and cheese are good sources of protein which is important for making muscle and other body tissue.

Have a helping of one or other of these foods at every meal—breakfast, lunch and supper.

There is no need to buy expensive meat as the cheaper cuts are equally nutritious. Vary your menu by using both white fish (e.g. cod) and oily fish (e.g. herrings, sardines), and eggs.

Meat (particularly liver, kidney, heart) and eggs are also good sources of *iron*. Iron is necessary not only for making and enriching your baby's blood, but also to prevent you becoming anaemic.
Try to put liver, kidney and heart, into your menu once or twice a week.

Vegetables

These provide vitamins necessary for baby's skin, eyes, and gums. Green vegetables also supply iron.
Have at least two helpings of vegetables or salad a day.
Buy vegetables in season. Boil in a small amount of water, until just cooked and serve immediately. Use the water left for making gravy or soup. Cooking and serving in this way helps to retain the vitamins.

Fruit

Fruit, like vegetables, provides vitamins. Fresh fruit should be eaten at least once a day.
Oranges, grapefruit and tomatoes are excellent sources of Vitamin C and should be included daily.

Cereals

Foods such as bread, potatoes, breakfast cereals, rice and semolina, provide bulk and variety to the diet as well as energy. Too much of these foods, however, leads to unnecessary increase in weight.

Fats

Some fats (such as butter and margarine) provide Vitamin A and D. Most cooking fats however do not.
If you choose your foods as suggested above, then your diet will adequately cover the increased requirements of pregnancy.

Note:

Foods such as sugar, jam, sweets, chocolates, cakes, biscuits, sweet drinks, pastry and fried foods contain very little food value, but many calories.

It is these foods which you should try to cut down or eliminate completely if you are gaining too much weight.

Problems

Below are some useful hints on how to prevent or alleviate some of the minor dietary problems which frequently occur during pregnancy.

Morning sickness

1. Have two plain biscuits but nothing to drink before rising.
2. Take your time in getting out of bed.
3. Have a light dry breakfast.
4. Introduce fluid slowly during the morning.

Heartburn and indigestion

1. Eat little and often instead of large meals.
2. Eat your meals slowly and chew food well.
3. Avoid fried, fatty and highly spiced foods.
4. Avoid drinking with your main meals.
5. Do not bend or lie down flat immediately after a meal.

Constipation

1. Eat some fresh fruit every day and some green vegetables or salad at mid-day and evening meals.
2. Have wholemeal bread or crispbread instead of white bread.
3. Try to drink plenty of water during the day.

If you need any further help—please ask your doctor to refer you to the dietitian.

With more concentration on group involvement in class, it would be difficult to give a talk exactly as above—apart from seeming didactic, attention would wander and perhaps very little of the content would be retained.

Some suggestions to make discussions of nutrition more attractive would be:
The use of a flannelgraph.

Actual food brought to class, with the group placing each item in its correct category, and talking about the content of 'made-up' and processed foods.

A day's diary of food brought along by each woman, for discussion of balance and nutritional value, or simply ticking categories of 'valuable' food she has eaten, to see how it compares with a balanced food plan for pregnancy displayed on an attractive poster. (Posters can be obtained from the Health Education Council, or made by the teacher herself from magazine cut-out pictures.)

A food 'quiz', prepared by the teacher, and marked by each group member for herself, so that she can test her awareness of good eating without being embarrassed by more knowledgeable members of the class.

Bright, simple leaflets, to take home after the discussion of nutrition. Some of these leaflets list categories of food, others give ideas for recipes.

Emotional changes

Thoughts, worries, attitude swings, sensitivity, changes in the relationships with husband and parents—these are all topics which might be discussed. The teacher may commence: 'One mother said, . . . do any of you feel like this?' 'Do you find you burst into tears easily?' 'What do you feel about the baby's movements?' 'What do your husbands say when the baby kicks them?' A question such as 'How many of you know that your husband wants to be present at the birth?' can lead to a general discussion of husbands' attitudes, and an invitation to bring them along to an evening class. When the group know each other well and are becoming freely vocal (perhaps after the first few weeks of meeting) a very revealing discussion can start with the question 'How many of you feel scared? Can you say why?' With practice and sensitivity a teacher can 'feel' how far a group wants to go in the exploration of their feelings.

Changes in life style and role

Under this heading might fall the following subjects: stopping work, loneliness, managing on one salary and budgeting, and difficulties with accommodation. Some mothers may feel 'different' and apart from their non-pregnant friends, and find subjects trivial which had been interesting, because the fact of pregnancy becomes all-absorbing.

Sexual relationships cause concern, both partners still needing warmth, reassurance, companionship and love. The teacher can introduce the subject by saying that some women become a great deal more sexually responsive in pregnancy, while others cannot respond as before—as if they were 'guarding' their bodies. In the same way, some men enjoy the greater sexual freedom of abandoning contraception, while others see their wives as the mother of their child, and are a little afraid of sexual activity. It is important to convey that neither attitude is 'wrong', but unresponsive wives could be encouraged by a reminder that sexual expression does not necessarily imply full intercourse, especially in very late pregnancy when it may be uncomfortable, but that loving caresses can be exchanged in many ways and different positions. Those teachers who have difficulty in discussing sexual matters in class may like to buy a new book by the American authors Elizabeth Bing and Libby Colman called *Making Love During Pregnancy* which is available in this country. It contains accounts of sexual feelings and activities during pregnancy, labour and the puerperium, from many articulate couples. It is illustrated by extremely frank but sensitively produced line drawings and would also be useful to lend to parents seeking information but too shy to talk about their needs.

Sharing the pregnancy with one's partner as much as possible should be stressed, talking about clinic visits, classes, moods and feelings.

Coping with difficulties

Here, the group can be encouraged to discuss freely anything which has bothered them during pregnancy, and how they, as a group, have found different ways of handling these difficulties.

For instance:

Vomiting and tiredness in early pregnancy

Increased irritability in the mucous linings of the body—vaginal irritations and discharge, excessive salivation, colds and coughs which 'hang on', catarrh

Cramp, indigestion, constipation, haemorrhoids, varicose veins

Stretch marks, backache

Difficulty in taking iron because of upsets of digestion

Being told old-wives' tales and horror stories

Sleeplessness

Pressure pains and nerve pains

Braxton-Hicks contractions strong enough to be painful

Waking in the night and feeling scared

'Going off sex'

Worries about the baby's normality—'We hear so much about things being wrong with babies these days. Are a lot of babies abnormal?'

Each discussion period will, of course, alter with the differentiation of age range, maturity, childbirth experiences, cultural level, and stage of pregnancy of the group. A widely differentiated group can be a very supportive one, although it is one which is more difficult for a teacher, as she is trying to 'give' different things to different members of it. Nevertheless, we have found that much of the 'giving' comes from individual members of the group, and that multigravidae often choose their words carefully, and give confidence to young primigravidae.

How can I remain comfortable, attractive, and regain my figure? (topic 4)

Some of these answers will be given in a talk or questions, or in group discussion, but in the third part of the class we aim at teaching body-awareness (see Teaching techniques, Ch. 2)—that is, to instil in the group the enthusiasm for regular practising of exercises, and day-to-day consciousness of their bodies and how they are using them.

Exercises should be taught with enthusiasm and care, encouraging the class to think of how their bodies are responding, and to appreciate the differences between tension and relaxation of different muscle groups, so that they become more aware of the action and reaction of their bodies in daily life, and in stress situations.

In the exercise session we would teach:

General relaxation

Preservative exercises for the abdominal wall, pelvic floor and breasts

Correct posture, when standing, sitting and walking

How to minimise strain when getting out of bed, lifting and carrying objects

Positions for rest which will prevent circulatory stasis.

This training will benefit every woman during pregnancy and afterwards, irrespective of the type of labour that she may have.

USEFUL EXPLANATIONS

Aiming always for simplicity and clarity, here are some suggestions of words to use when giving a set talk, answering direct questions in group discussion, and teaching neuromuscular control and awareness. It is neither possible nor necessary, in a book of this size, to describe all the talks and discussions in full. We have therefore chosen a few topics which, in our experience, many teachers find difficult to portray simply. It is not our intention that these words should be followed slavishly—they are given merely as examples for teachers to consider.

A new teacher should not be afraid of simplicity. In a mixed class many will have studied biology at school, but during pregnancy an easily understood and emotionally satisfying explanation is more appropriate for almost all intelligence levels.

The pelvis and pelvic floor

Visual aids: drawings or film slides, and model pelvis held against the teacher's body as she talks.

'As you can see, the pelvis is an irregular circle of bone at the bottom of the body, and this model looks like one solid bone. There are two main bones which meet at the front here and are joined together at the base of the spine by a third triangular-shaped bone, the sacrum. Below the sacrum are four small bones called the coccyx which in animals extend to form the tail.' (The class can then feel the dimples on either side of the base of the spine which indicate the sacro-iliac joints, the hip promontories, and the symphysis pubis.) 'These four bones have joints here which relax a little in pregnancy. The baby's head' (demonstrated with a model) 'has to go through this circle, and in a first pregnancy it usually lies right inside it before labour begins. When that happens your doctor says the head is "engaged". After the first pregnancy the abdominal muscles can stretch more and the baby has more room to move so doesn't need to have its head "engaged" until labour begins.

'Pelvis is a Latin word meaning basin—but you can see this basin hasn't got a bottom. The bottom of the basin is a sling of muscles called the pelvic floor—layers of muscles covering this area here. From the front to the back, underneath your body, it has three openings, the front one leads to the bladder, the middle one is the vagina or birth canal and the back one leads to the bowel. One purpose of these muscles is to support all the organs of the pelvis. They also have important strengthening bands in them; one makes a complete ring round the back passage and another a loop which is attached by its ends to the arch of bone in front and surrounds the two front passages. The purpose of these bands is to control what passes in and out of this part of the body.

'We shall be learning especially how to appreciate the control of these muscles, but you all know how to control them to some extent already—how to tighten the muscles round the bladder opening and the bowel opening when either of them are full, and how to relax the muscles to empty the bladder or to have your bowels opened when it's convenient to do so. In the same way, you know how to relax the vagina to admit your husband's penis, and then how to tense and relax it when making love.' (This can be a good opportunity to stop and discuss sex in pregnancy, if the class seems receptive.) 'In the practical part of the class we shall build up greater control of these muscles, so that they will be strengthened to take the extra weight during pregnancy, be able to relax to let the baby be born, and then recover well from their stretching afterwards.'

Routine antenatal examinations

The group will have been having routine examinations for some time before attending the classes, and these can profitably be discussed.

'Each antenatal visit includes the testing of a specimen of urine, recording blood pressure, and measuring the height of the womb or uterus. At some time there will be at least one vaginal examination, and at least one specimen of blood taken for examination. Later on in pregnancy the baby's heart-beat is counted at each visit and the position of the baby recorded.'

It is worthwhile to ascertain how many of the class have 'cooperation cards'. In some areas these are used when a general practitioner and a hospital share the responsibility of antenatal care. Each patient keeps her own card, in an unsealed envelope, and all examinations are recorded on it. This is an easy way of conveying information between the hospital and family doctor, but appears to cause additional stress to the pregnant woman. She, of course, reads as much of her notes as she can interpret—it would take superhuman restraint not to do so, as she wishes to obtain reassurance that everything is going well. Instead of this, she worries about the meanings of the abbreviations on the card. As one woman said, 'I look at my card and, if it says the same thing each week, I don't worry, but I've been worried all week'. Instead of 'Vx' her doctor had written 'cephal' so she only needed to be told that the terms were virtually exchangeable. We feel that all antenatal teachers should be familiar with abbreviated terms, and be able to show the recorded position of the baby with a model against her own body.

However, antenatal clinics are changing, and women are being given more information about themselves. We see no reason why all the records should not be available to the pregnant mother—pregnancy is not an illness.

There are, in many branches of medicine, valid reasons for shielding a patient from her records. For instance, a woman with a malignancy may be devastated if she read of the extent of her illness, just at the time when her morale and buoyant optimism would be needed as one of the most essential factors of her treatment.

But a pregnant woman is looking after her child herself. She is the most important member of the team which is maintaining that child's health.

Medical opinion supports the view that a woman should be told as much as possible. In the antenatal clinic, all staff have been asked to work to maintain 'emotional wellbeing' as well as physical health (see Report of Working Party on Antenatal Care, pp. 11–12). Some hospitals are trusting women to carry all their records from one area of the clinic to other departments, and explaining to each patient how their pregnancy is progressing.

Some women have complained that after a very long wait, they only see a doctor for few seconds, and there is no opportunity for conversation (Boyd & Sellers, 1982). This is inevitable because of the pressure of work carried by consultants and registrars in a busy maternity unit. This difficulty is resolved by seeing a senior midwife, and discussing the records with her, after she has seen the doctor.

Together they check what has been written. If the baby is in an unusual position—for instance a transverse lie or a breech—the midwife will explain what is likely to happen at this stage. If the woman wishes, she can listen to the baby's heartbeats with a Sonic Aid.

She then goes home feeling that somebody cares, has time, and that she has been treated as an individual.

Where this does not happen, or when the midwives are busy with others and the woman cannot wait, she will, as formerly, ask all her questions at the antenatal class.

Ideally, the class teaching will be shared by a midwife who is in contact with the mother's own hospital, and knows what would have been said at the antenatal clinic.

If this is not so, it is important that the class teacher knows the hospitals and their routine procedures. She should also, ideally, have the confidence of the staff, and feel a member of the team.

She then (whether health visitor or obstetric physiotherapist) can answer any questions honestly and with validity.

If a teacher does not know the answer to any question, or the policy of the hospital or midwife, she should be able to contact them to discuss any problem, so that the mother can be reassured very shortly.

Thus morale and emotional health can be maintained by the cooperation of all who are caring, in any way, for each mother.

Some ways of talking about antenatal tests are as follow:

Urine testing and pre-eclampsia. 'The urine specimen has two main functions. The first is to check that no sugar is present. Sometimes, mild diabetes is discovered in pregnancy and special care with diet will be needed. The second is to check that no albumin (or protein) is in the urine. This could come from contamination by a vaginal discharge, which should be discussed with the doctor and may need treatment. The albumin is more important when it is in the urine itself, as it means that the kidneys are letting the protein into the urine instead of passing it to the rest of the body, and may be a sign of pre-eclampsia. Nobody quite knows why this begins, but it appears that the body is becoming tired of carrying the baby and at the same time living a normal busy life. The kidneys start to work inefficiently and besides letting protein slip through, they don't get rid of enough water so that there is a fairly large weight gain of fluid, usually starting in the feet and ankles. The technical name for this gathering of fluid is oedema. Then the blood pressure starts to rise, and the doctor will order a woman to rest, and sometimes prescribe sedatives, or medicine to get rid of the fluid. In pre-eclampsia it is essential to rest as much as the doctor recommends, and he may also advise a salt-restricted diet. However, from the beginning of pregnancy a woman can help herself to remain healthy by restricting her salt, being careful not to overeat, especially starchy foods, and being sensible about resting part of each day.'

Preventing abortions

Women are rightly becoming more familiar with obstetric terms as they assume more rights over their own bodies, so a woman in class may mention that she has a Shirodkar suture round her cervix. This can be described as a draw-string not unlike the fastening of the home-made old-fashioned 'dolly' bags, and that it is done, under anaesthetic, when a woman has already had one abortion, and the obstetrician feels that the reason may have been a cervix which dilates easily (an incompetent cervix). By tightening the cervix during pregnancy, this is overcome, and the stitch can be removed at the end of pregnancy. Normally, other tests are performed, one of which is a simple smear, taken from the vagina to assess hormone balance. If progesterone is found to be deficient, a course of hormone treatments is given, usually by injection, to correct the imbalance.

We have known instances when during discussion, women have talked about the treatment given to them to save their baby, and have used a description very similar to the above, to the interest of the other mothers, who have from then followed the successful progress of the pregnancy with great pleasure.

An early blood specimen. 'This is taken for several reasons:

'First, to find the blood group, in case at any time a woman needs a blood transfusion, but this is a rare thing to happen.

'Second, to see how much iron is in the blood. The baby takes a lot of iron, especially at the end of pregnancy, and if a woman's body is short of iron she will feel very tired and faint, be anaemic and generally miserable. That's why when iron is prescribed it is important to keep taking it regularly. If one type produces discomforts—tummy pains, constipation or diarrhoea—another sort can be tried. No woman should stop taking iron because of these upsets, but let her doctor know. However, iron is much easier to digest if taken with a protein meal.' (It is useful here to discuss protein foods, and also foods rich in iron—liver, kidney, dried fruit, cocoa, egg yolks.)

'The third important discovery in the blood specimen is the Rh or Rhesus factor. If a woman is Rhesus negative and her husband Rhesus positive, the baby may be positive too; than the baby's blood will be different from the mother's. The afterbirth, or placenta, which is passing food to the baby and waste material back to the mother, acts as a partial barrier between the mother's and baby's blood, like a sieve so that food can be exchanged without the blood mixing. However, sometimes a few blood cells get through the placenta to the mother, and her blood forms antibodies to them, because they are different, just like it would form antibodies to an infection. With good modern care this Rh factor is becoming less important. The time when the placental barrier works least well is in labour, so with the first child antibodies are rarely a problem.'

External version

'This is a fairly common manoeuvre, usually carried out in hospital. If the examining doctor finds that the baby, instead of coming head

first, is bumping its head against your ribs, in the breech position'
(demonstrate with a doll) 'he may try to push the baby into a head
first position. This is not a painful experience, as he applies gentle
pressure. First, he asks you to lie back and relax, then with one
hand on the baby's head through your abdominal muscles, and a
hand guiding its bottom, he strokes the baby round to a head first
position, in the direction of the curve of the baby's spine.

'This is attempted at about 34–35 weeks of pregnancy, because if
it is done too early, the baby might just flip back again to the position he is used to lying in. If tried too late, the baby may be too large
to turn.

'In the past, doctors would have several attempts at this
manoeuvre, sometimes giving a sedative to aid relaxation. Today,
it is usual after one attempt, if the baby is still in "breech" position,
to deliver it like this, or consider a Caesarean section, as these are
becoming much more common and very safe.'

Fetal monitoring in pregnancy

Monitoring of the fetus in pregnancy has become much more sophisticated so that the baby's condition in the uterus can be more accurately observed than ever before, and premature labour often
averted.

Together, ultrasound, heart monitoring, and maternal blood
sampling for human placental lactogen and oestriol, can provide an
accurate picture of the baby's progress, which can be plotted and
easily followed on charts and electrocardiograms.

If a baby is thought to be 'at risk'—the many reasons could
include small growth for dates, any haemorrhage from the uterus,
pre-eclampsia and diabetes—the mother can be admitted into
hospital or seen in outpatients clinic, and the baby observed.

One of these ways is fetal heart monitoring. 'What is this?'

'For a long time, in labour, a sensitive microphone has been used
to record the baby's heartbeat. The microphone is placed on your
abdomen, fastened with a comfortable elastic band, and the machine
then records a pattern on paper of the baby's heartbeat. Also a light
flashes in the machine to the rhythm of the heart. Now that
hospitals have more machines available, they can be used in the
antenatal wards too.

'There are lots of causes of going into hospital before labour, and
you will always have an opportunity to discuss with the doctor why
you should come in early. Sometimes it is only for a few days rest,
and you are sent home again.

'To be sure that the baby is doing well, some hospitals record the baby's heartbeat for a few minutes each day, sometimes "jogging" the baby a little while the machine is working, by moving your abdomen as if they were examining you. The baby's heartbeat is steady and then changes rhythm when this movement is done, and the staff know that the baby is healthy.

The 'kick chart' (Cardiff count-to-ten fetal activity chart). This is a simple way in which a mother monitors her own baby. Some hospitals give each patient a kick chart, towards the end of pregnancy, which is rather like a temperature chart to look at, divided into days and hours. Beginning from 9 a.m. each movement of the baby is marked, with the time it occurs, until ten movements have been recorded. At the bottom of the chart are instructions: 'If you feel less than 10 movements on 2 consecutive days, or if you feel *no* movements during one day, please phone us.'

Lack of movements can mean that the baby is just asleep, but, to be sure, the Midwifery Nursing Officer will ask you to come in, so that you can both listen to the baby's heartbeat with the Sonic Aid machine, or the abdominal monitoring band.

'Another way of fetal monitoring is to see that the placenta is working well by taking a little of your blood to examine. This can be done in outpatients, but if you are in hospital it is done once or twice a week. Two substances are measured—both hormones—from the one specimen of blood, and the doctor can be sure that the placenta is growing and nourishing the baby adequately.

'One of these hormones can also be measured in urine, but to get an accurate figure, a whole day's specimens of urine have to be saved. In the past, women used to be going up to hospital carrying large bottles of their 24 hours' collection. Again, a blood specimen is simpler and more accurate.'

Premature labour. 'Even with all this care, labour may start too early. It is possible now, in many cases, to stop the labour by injections. If it seems that, even with the injections, the baby is going to be born soon, a substance can be given to the mother to help her baby's lungs to develop, and so to function better at birth.

'As you can see, babies today are protected and monitored better than ever before, throughout pregnancy, and more mature and healthier babies are being born.'

Ultrasonic echo sounding (ultrasound), sometimes called a 'scan'

In the 1950s and early 1960s this technique of echo-sounding was being developed in Glasgow University by Professor Ian Donald. His work was inspired by the echo-sounding for submarines in the

1939–45 war, which recorded density, and produced a picture on a cathode-ray screen. A sound probe of high frequency, above that of the human ear, records density in the abdomen and when the whole abdomen has been stroked by the probe, and processed through a computer, a picture is produced which can be photographed and preserved. At first, very few research workers were skilled enough to interpret this with accuracy, but many more have now been trained, and this screening procedure should be available to any pregnant woman. If a small maternity hospital does not possess its own equipment, the woman will be referred to the nearest hospital with an ultrasound machine, and the findings will be sent to her hospital.

This technique is particularly useful as much can be learned about the fetus and its surroundings, there is no pain, and no known harmful effects to mother or baby.

It is replacing X-rays to a large extent as a diagnostic aid, as more can be learned than by an ordinary X-ray.

It can diagnose pregnancy as early as three weeks after conception, diagnose twins at a very early stage, and accurately measure the size of the baby's head or body, throughout pregnancy, if there is doubt about dates or the baby's growth. The position of the placenta can be located, in cases of suspected placenta praevia, or before an amniocentesis (see below).

One of the latest machines is the 3-D scanner, which produces a three-dimensional picture of the baby. Even fingers, and individual bones of the spine, can be photographed.

Now that the ultrasound scan is becoming one of the frequent ways of measuring and monitoring the baby's progress, the teacher will probably be told by a class member that she has just had the investigation. Some of the class will not have heard of it, so a simple explanation can be given, together, if she wishes, with the class member describing what it felt like. She will have been given the reason for the scan, such as 'We want to find where the afterbirth is', or 'Let's see if you're having twins', or maybe 'The baby's a bit small, we're going to keep measuring the growth of it's head'. If she hasn't fully understood the reason, she should be encouraged to ask for more information on her next visit.

In fact, in many hospitals now, the routine is for each pregnant woman to have at least one ultrasonic scan during her pregnancy. It is useful to explain this procedure, therefore, in an 'early pregnancy' class—by late pregnancy it will be already familiar. A simple explanation would be:

'You will lie comfortably on your back on a bed. Your abdomen will be covered all over with oil. A large machine will be over the bed, and a small crystal which is attached to the machine will glide over the oil, up and down and from side to side. The only discomfort will be that you will be asked not to empty your bladder beforehand, as a full bladder gives a better picture, and it's a bit uncomfortable to be lying waiting to go to the lavatory. Apart from this, the only sensation will be one of touch. The sound which is transmitted is above the range of the human ear so you will hear nothing, but echoes of the sound waves trace a picture on a screen. This can show the size and position of both the baby and the placenta.'

Amniocentesis

The technique of obtaining a small sample of amniotic fluid by paracentesis through the abdominal wall is being used more frequently today, and gives much information in certain cases. The alphafetoprotein level can be accurately measured (see below) and in Rhesus incompatibility the amount of bilirubin in the liquor can determine the baby's condition, because a high amount of bilirubin indicates excessive breakdown of fetal red blood cells. Fortunately Rhesus incompatibility is becoming rare today, as since the 1940s great care has been taken in matching blood for Rh factors in transfusions. The first baby is rarely affected, as the baby's Rhesus positive cells appear not to enter the mother's blood stream until labour. A test of the blood from the baby's cord, if Rhesus negative, is then made, to determine the amount of positive cells which have entered her circulation. All Rhesus negative women with Rhesus positive babies are then given an injection of anti-D immunoglobulin within 2–3 days. This destroys the fetal positive cells and prevents the formation of antibodies which could affect further babies.

This anti-D immunoglobulin is also given after an abortion or planned termination, if positive cells are found in the woman's body. (Termination of pregnancy is not considered lightly, and one consequence, before this monitoring, is that a woman who has had a record of abortions or terminations may already have Rh antibodies in her blood during her first full-term pregnancy.) The sex of the baby can be identified and this is important if the parents carry genes of sex-linked congenital disorders. Towards term it can also estimate the maturity of the fetus, as sebaceous activity begins in the skin in late pregnancy, and this activity can be shown by staining the cells. Estimation of the lecithin/sphingomyelin ratio in the cells of the amniotic fluid also measures maturity, and the liquor may be tested for this before an induction, to make sure that the lungs are sufficiently developed for delivery.

One would normally not mention this in class, but if a question is asked about it one could say:

'Yes, sometimes the liquor that the baby is floating in is examined by inserting a needle through the abdomen after a local anaesthetic has been given. It is still a fairly rare procedure as complicated laboratory tests are carried out on the liquor withdrawn, and as yet there is not enough staff or money to do this often. If, for instance, a woman had given birth to one damaged child, and genetic analysis had shown that there were high risks of further abnormalities, she could have this procedure and the doctors would know for certain whether or not she was carrying a child with certain severe abnormalities. If she wasn't, there would be great relief for the rest of the pregnancy. If she was, an abortion might be offered. This can apply to other rare conditions also. If the examination of the liquor were a quick, easy and cheap thing to do, it could be done in late pregnancy to find out if the mother's dates were correct, as the maturity of the fetus could be estimated by examining the cells and chemical substances in the liquor.'

Alphafetoprotein measurements

In the late 1960s amniocentesis was becoming more common, and the fluid obtained was mainly used for cell examination. In Edinburgh, at the Department of Human Genetics at Western General Hospital, Professor Alan Emery was becoming more interested in the fluid itself. He concentrated on substances occurring in amniotic fluid, especially proteins and enzymes. Soon the work concentrated on alphafetoprotein, present in a fetus but not an adult, and secreted by the fetus into the amniotic fluid.

In long experimentation, the amount of alphafetoprotein secreted by a normal fetus was plotted, and in 1972 it was discovered that a baby with an open spina bifida, or anencephaly, had a very significant rise of this serum protein. This was printed in *The Lancet* in July of that year. From then, it was possible to diagnose these conditions when the pregnancy was in a fairly early stage, and termination was possible.

Women 'at risk' especially those with previously deformed children, were offered this test, although their views on termination, should the test be positive, were discussed carefully first. With strong views against termination the test loses its validity.

Shortly afterwards, it was discovered that some alphafetoprotein entered the mother's blood circulation, and a specimen of blood from the mother, taken between the 16th and 18th weeks of pregnancy, could show a significant rise, if these deformities, or twins, were being carried. This blood test is now routine for women 'at risk' of a deformed child.

Some hospitals have gone further, and are testing blood specimens of all pregnant women for alphafetoprotein (or AFP). An explanation could be as follows:

'It is now the routine of the hospital to take a specimen of blood from each woman between the 16th and 18th weeks of pregnancy. This tests for a substance called alphafetoprotein, and can alert for the presence of twins, or some abnormalities, such as spina bifida. You will not be notified if the blood specimen is normal. Should it show a raised level, you will be notified, and asked to give a second blood specimen. If this is also raised, you will talk to the doctor, who will explain further tests. An ultrasound scan will show twins or triplets, for example, and will identify the length of the pregnancy, as, if the blood tests are taken at the wrong time, an inaccurate reading is shown.

'If the reading seems accurate, amniocentesis is performed. You will remember that the scan is always done before the amniocentesis, so that the doctor knows the position of the baby and the placenta, and there is no danger of touching them. As you know already, lots of things can be found by examining this fluid—cells floating in it identify the sex of the baby, in Rhesus incompatibility the baby's condition can be estimated and of course the alphafetoprotein can be accurately measured, which can show up some abnormalities of the baby.

'If the baby was found to be imperfect, which is extremely unlikely, the husband and wife would be counselled carefully together and their views on termination respected. If a damaged child is suspected, the amniocentesis is performed as quickly as possible, as this, of course, is a very anxious time for the parents.'

Amnioscopy

Again, this is rare, but an amnioscope can be passed through the cervix and the colour and, to a certain extent, amount of liquor can be assessed. If asked about this the reply could be that the doctor, by this examination, can estimate the baby's condition if he thinks all is not going well, as the liquor changes colour if the baby gets distressed.

NEUROMUSCULAR CONTROL IN PREGNANCY

Each time exercises are taught it should be stressed that some of them can be practised while carrying out everyday tasks, for instance pelvic floor control can be practised sitting at an office desk, waiting for a bus, or washing up, so that the idea is firmly implanted that practising should not be restricted to just once a day, but done several times every day. We are trying to teach each woman to notice some of the hundreds of sensations which arise in her muscles and joints, to register them in her brain, and to transmit appropriate responses to other muscles and joints. For example, before we can improve a woman's posture, we must first make her aware of what she is doing with the different parts of her body. Only then can we teach her to modify the position of her head, the tilt of her pelvis, and so forth. Similarly, no woman will learn to relax at will until she can appreciate the different 'feel' of tense and relaxed muscles. It is a question of applying mental concentration rather than physical effort to appreciate this body-awareness, and some people find it more difficult than others. An analogy can be made in class of the conscious muscle-coordination needed to ride a bicycle or to swim, and how hard one had to think of one's arms and legs and balance. With practice the body begins to work in harmony until one acquires the art of cycling or swimming and can go on doing it quite automatically while thinking of something else.

The class should begin practising after using the toilets and removing constricting clothes. Tights, slacks or pyjama trousers save any embarrassment, and the teacher should also wear tights or slacks and be prepared to demonstrate.

The exercises described below cover only the basic minimum; an experienced physiotherapist would include a good deal more. Readers are referred to books and pamphlets by McLaren (1973), Montgomery (1969) and Williams (1969).

To tone the muscles supporting the breasts. Get the mothers to sit in a comfortable position on their mattresses, not supported by pillows, then proceed as follows:

'Clasp your hands together, palms touching, fingers upwards, and elbows at right-angles to the body, about shoulder height. Press your hands together as hard as possible—harder—hold it—relax. Remain in the same position, now repeat the pressure—harder—hold it—and relax.'

The teacher should check that the class really does feel the 'lift' at each side of the chest.

Breath control. The women are asked to put their hands on their lower ribs (or just above their vanished waistline). The teacher's request then is, 'Breathe out, feel your fingers coming together. Now let your chest fill with air again and notice how your hands are pushed apart'. While they are breathing in this controlled fashion the teacher should watch that they are breathing easily and regularly, and discourage them from trying too hard, probably saying something like, 'Just gentle, easy, deep breathing, to your own rhythm'.

To strengthen abdominal muscles, combined with pelvic rocking. The women are asked to lie down on their backs, heads and necks well supported and knees bent.

'You are now going to pull your tummy in so that you pull the baby towards your backbone and at the same time press your backbone to the floor. Ready—pull—in, let—go. Notice the different sensations. Did you feel how your pelvis tilted up in front when you flattened your backs, and tilted down when you relaxed and your backs hollowed a little?' (The teacher can demonstrate by moving the model pelvis or a basin, at the same time rocking her own pelvis, and the class can feel their hip promontories moving when they do the exercise.) 'This is called pelvic rocking and can be done in lots of different positions, lying on the side, sitting or standing. This exercise keeps your tummies from getting overstretched and helps to relieve the kind of backache which you get from sitting or lying too long in one position. Practising relaxation of the tummy muscles will enable the doctor or midwife to feel the baby's head more easily and give you less discomfort when they are examining you'.

Relaxation (Modified Jacobsen's method)

This is one method of becoming aware of tension and its release. The women lie on their backs, heads and shoulders well supported, and a pillow or bolster under their knees so that they are slightly bent. The teacher should check that she can see all the class and that they are all comfortable. When satisfied with this she can begin.

'Now you are going to learn how to relax. Just bend your right elbow a little—stop bending it and let go. Notice that your muscles feel different when they are pulling from when they stop pulling and let go—that is, relax. Try again, but this time tighten the arm muscles without actually moving, as if you were going to bend your elbow. Relax the muscles, put your other hand on your upper arm and feel the difference. Feel that your arm is heavy, resting and comfortable. Now the shoulder muscles. Lift your arm away from your body, and let it fall. Tighten the muscles without lifting, let them relax, feel comfortable and notice the difference in sensations.

'Now tighten your shoulder, elbow, wrist and hand so that your whole arm feels hard and tense. Let go. Repeat with the other arm. Tighten the muscles of one leg, let go. Repeat with the other one. Tighten your tummy muscles, let go. Hollow your back so that the two columns of muscle on either side of your spine stand out in hard ridges. Let go and feel your spine go slack as if you are resting in an old deck chair. Screw up your face in a horrible grimace, let go and feel the tension going from your mouth, your eyes and your forehead so that all the lines disappear and your face has no expression.

'Notice that you tend to hold your breath when you go tense and breathe out when you relax. Now, breathe in, hold your breath and make your whole body rigid, give a big sigh out and let the tension flow out of your arms, legs, bodies and faces. Breathe a little more slowly and deeply than usual, just enough to make you think about the rhythm of your breathing, and each time you breathe out try to get rid of a little bit more tension.'

When the class are able to appreciate their widely differing sensations when they are in a state of complete tension followed by complete relaxation, the teacher can ask them to move a little, then simply to breathe in, out and relax completely without any preliminary tension so that they can learn to differentiate between the normal slight movements and tensions and complete controlled relaxation.

The women are then asked to turn on their sides and to repeat the exercises. Some will like to have their lower arm extended behind them, others are more comfortable with it underneath them. In any case they should have their upper leg bent more than the lower one, so that both legs can rest and the abdomen is partially supported by the mattress. More pillows may be needed under the abdomen and upper leg.

Teachers are referred to Eileen Montgomery's book *At Your Best for Birth and Later* for a more detailed description of this method of teaching relaxation.

Later, special effort should be spent on the pelvic floor, so that each member of the class becomes aware of the sensation of tightening and relaxing the muscles round the anus, and the urethra and bladder. The anal sphincter is the easiest to control, so the women are asked to imagine the ring of muscle deep inside the back passage and to tighten this ring so that the passage closes. Control of the vaginal sphincter can be learned simply at first. 'You're on top of a bus and longing to go to the lavatory. Pull in underneath. Now let go. Feel that the muscles have become softer, with no resistance.' If some are not sure of the sensation they can be asked to try occasionally, when their bladders are full, to stop a flow of urine in midstream, record the sensation of tightening, then feel the release as they begin to urinate again. They can also be encouraged to tighten the whole muscle sling as if going up in a lift, slowly, one floor at a time, getting extra tightness floor by floor until the fifth or sixth floor is reached, then slowly down, releasing a little more at each floor until the ground floor is passed and the basement is reached with awareness of complete relaxation. The class is then asked to tighten a little, as if reaching the ground floor again and to leave the muscles in their normal state of tone. The muscles of the thighs and buttocks should not be brought into play.

During the exercises for pelvic floor control the teacher can discuss how a relaxed vagina makes a vaginal examination more comfortable. The class can be asked to practise relaxing 'towards' the doctor's fingers by breathing out and allowing their pelvic floor to feel the maximum 'basement' type relaxation and their thighs to fall outwards, then to breathe gently and shallowly in their upper chests as the doctor inserts his fingers. The teacher can also explain the importance of this examination—how it is sometimes used to confirm the pregnancy, but is mainly to estimate the size of the opening in the pelvic basin. Some women have been perturbed to see a doctor's fist approaching their pelvic floor, only to find that the fist is simply pressed against the muscles. The size of the pelvic opening can be estimated by this simple manoeuvre also.

After the tension and release exercises the class should not be left for more than a few minutes to rest. We are teaching muscle control and are not anxious to encourage sleep. The class should, however, get up very slowly, as after even a short period of relaxation, quick activity can cause dizziness. So the teacher continues thus:

'Take a few deep breaths, then pretend you are large tabby cats in a patch of sunshine. Stretch, luxuriate, and wriggle until you are ready to get up. Then, if on your side, put your top hand on the floor, push up first with this hand and then with your other hand until you are kneeling on all-fours. Change to half-kneeling with one foot on the ground, then stand up. If you had been lying on your back, you would have bent your knees, rolled over, and then come up from a side position to avoid strain on the tummy muscles.'

Correct posture

With the class standing—

'Let me see how you stand when you are tired. Now get a good standing position instead of slouching, grow as tall as possible, feel as if you are being pulled upwards by a string through the crown of your head, keep your bustline in front of your tummy. Brace your tummy and tail muscles slightly as if you are wearing a good belt. Adjust your balance so that your weight falls evenly between the heels and balls of your feet. Take a look in the mirror when you are standing like this, and notice how much better you look.'

Similarly the women's sitting positions are checked. The teacher then demonstrates wrong and right ways of picking up objects from the floor and the class then practises.

'Show me how you would pick a pin up from the floor. Bend your knees with one foot a little in front of the other, legs a little apart. Keep your back straight. Pick up the pin, straighten the knees and rise up. If you want to pick up a bucket or basket with one hand, stand close to it with the foot opposite to the hand with which you are going to lift, in front.'

The class practises with pillows.

At the end of the exercise session the class is reminded of each exercise, asked to practise several times a day and to think about their muscles, so that they become aware of their body sensation when not practising.

TIMING OF TEACHING ABOUT PREGNANCY

The talk about pregnancy, and exercises for pregnancy, are given as early as possible. Some teachers are able to arrange a class very early, shortly after the pregnancy is confirmed, but most will find that this teaching has to be given in the initial class of the set series, i.e., during the third trimester. Group discussion on thoughts and feelings, adjustments and difficulties, will continue throughout the course, however, and there is no attempt to confine this discussion on pregnancy to the initial classes. The women want reassurance about what is happening *now*, and as they get to know each other, and lose inhibitions, the discussion develops week by week, following different patterns in each course.

AIDS FOR MOTHERS AND BABIES

Since our last edition, the NCT has formed a limited company for the sale of goods useful to expectant and nursing mothers. These include, for the mother, 3 types of Mava bra, nightdresses of different patterns, a slip suitable for nursing, stretch briefs for holding sanitary towels and nursing nipple shields. For the baby there are suits, baby nests, holdalls. They can also give details of two baby carriers which they recommend, the 'Kangourou' and the 'Snuggli'.

With the exception of the carriers all these goods can be ordered by post or bought from the NCT (Maternity Sales Ltd), 9 Queensborough Terrace London W2, Telephone 01 221 3833. A catalogue and order form will be sent on request.

Support tights

Can be ordered on prescription from local chemist
Also available:

Elbeo maternity support tights 2 deniers	Selfridges Oxford Street LondonW1
Mothercare maternity tights	Branches of Mothercare and by post.

REFERENCES

Asians in Britain (1976) Public Relations Department, Van den Berghs & Jurgens Ltd, Sussex House, Civic Way, Burgess Hill, Sussex.

Beattie, J. (1981) Fetal Alcohol Syndrome–the incurable hangover. *Health Visitor*, 468–469.

Boyd, C., Sellers L. (1982) *The British Way of Birth*. London: Pan Books.

British Medical Journal (1978) 2, Nov. 11th p. 1317

Craddock, D. (1978) *Obesity and its Management*, p. 143–159. Edinburgh: Churchill Livingstone.

Department of Health and Social Service (1973) *Recommended Intakes of Nutrients for the United Kingdom*. London: HMSO.

Department of Health and Social Security (1978) *Eating for Health*, p. 161. London: HMSO.

Mackay, B. *Obstetrics and the Newborn*. London: Saunders.

Maternity Care in Action. (1982) Part 1. Ante-natal care. London: Maternity Services Advisory Committee.

Montgomery, E. (1969) *At Your Best for Birth and Later*, pp. 28–38. Bristol: Wright.

Reid, R. (1977) *My Children, My Children*, (Life before and after birth—an account of some recent developments). London: BBC Publications.

Winter, G. B. (1976) Maternal nutritional requirements in relation to the subsequent development of teeth in children, *Journal of Human Nutrition*, **30**, No. 2, 93.

World Health Organisation Committee (1965) *Nutrition in Pregnancy and Lactation*, WHO Report Service, 302.

Wyn, A. & Wyn, M. (1972) *Some Consequences of Induced Abortion to Children Born Subsequently*. Foundation for Education and Research into Childbearing, 27 Walpole Street, London SW3.

FOR FURTHER READING

Bing, E. & Colman, L. (1978) *Making Love During Pregnancy*, London: Bantam Books.

Birch, K., Chambers, M. (1982) *So you want to be a parent? The A.B.C. of feelings*. London: Richardson-Vicks.

Bloom, A. (1975) *Diabetes Explained*. London: Medical Technical Publishing.

Bourne, G. (1972) *Pregnancy*. London: Cassell.

Close, S. (1972) *The Know-How of Pregnancy and Labour*, Bristol: Wright.

Close, S. (1980) *The Toddler and the New Baby*. London: Routledge & Kegan Paul.

Colman, A. & Colman, L. (1971) *Pregnancy—The Psychological Experience*. New York: Herder & Herder.

Davidson, S., Passmore, R., Brock, J. F. & Truswell, A. (1979) *Human Nutrition and Dietetics*. Edinburgh: Churchill Livingstone.

Edwards, G. (1983) Alcohol and advice to the Pregnant Woman. *British Medical Journal* **286**, 247–8

Hungerford, M. J. (1972) *Childbirth Education*. Springfield, Illinois: Thomas.

Kitzinger, S. (1971) *Sex in Pregnancy* and *Sex After Baby*, Reprints from *Mother and Baby* obtained from NCT.

Laurence, K. M., James, N., Miller, M., Campbell, H. (1980) Increased risk of recurrence of pregnancies complicated by fetal neural tube defects in mothers receiving poor diets, and possible benefits of dietary counselling. *British Medical Journal*, **281**, 1593–1594.

Lewis, C. (ed.) (1982) *Growing Up with Good Food*. London: Unwin.

Liddell, C. (1977) *Mother's Superdiet—Healthy Eating for You and Your Baby*. Nickey Ross, London: Pitman.

Little, R., Streissguth, A. (1980) Prevention of fetal alcohol syndrome. *Alcoholism: Clinical and Experimental Research* **4**, 2.

Llewellyn-Jones, D. (1978) *Everywoman*, 2nd edn. London: Faber & Faber.

Loader, A. (ed.) (1980) *Pregnancy & Parenthood*. Oxford: Oxford University Press for the NCT.

Macintyre, S. (1977) *Single and Pregnant*, Crown Holm Ltd.

Macfarlane, A. (1977) *The Psychology of Childbirth*. London: Fontana.

Madders, J. (1980) *Stress and Relaxation*. London: Martin Dumitz.

Maternity Center Association (1968) *Guide for Expectant Parents*, New York. Obtainable from MCA, 48 East 92nd Street, New York 10028.

Mclaren, J. (1977) *Preparation for Parenthood—Notes for use with Antenatal Classes*, packs of 50. London: Murray.

Noble, E. (1980) (English edition) *Essential Exercises for the Childbearing Year*. London: Murray.

Oakley, A. (1981) *From Here to Maternity—Becoming a Mother*. London: Pelican.

Perkins, E. (1980) *Education for Childbirth and Parenthood*. London: Croom Helm.

Pitt, B. (1978) *Feelings about Childbirth*. London: Sheldon Press.

Rayner, C. (1977) *Claire Rayner Answers your 100 Questions on Pregnancy*. London: BBC Publications.

Rosen, M. G. & Rosen, L. (1977) *Your Baby's Brain Before Birth*. New York: Plume Books.

Shepherd, R. J. (1982) *The Risks of Passive Smoking*. London: Croom Helm.

Smithells, R. W. et al (1981) Vitamin supplementation and neural tube defects. *Lancet*, ii, 1425.

Sumiko, 1981, *My Baby Brother Ned*. London: Heinemann.

Verny, T., Kelly, J. (1982) *The Secret Life of the Unborn Child*. London: Sphere Books.

Weiss, J. S. (1981) *Your Second Child*. London: Sphere Books.

Coming shortly *Miscarriage*, National Childbirth Trust.

Some leaflets and booklets—most of them freely available to clinics

A Healthy Pregnancy. In English, Bengali, Gujarati, Hindi, Punjabi, and Urdu. Health Education Council, 78 New Oxford Street, London W1. A very attractive new booklet illustrated with pictures of different Indian mothers.

Expectant Parents (1978) National Association for Maternal & Child Welfare, 1 South Audley Street London W1Y 6JS.

Your First Baby (1980) The Royal College of Midwives. Newbourne Group Publications, 91 Stoke Newington Church Street, London N16 OAU.

A Guide for the Expectant Mother (1980) National Dairy Council, John Princes Street, London WIM OAP.

How to Help Yourself to Have a Healthy Baby. The Spastics Society, 12 Park Crescent, London WIN 4EQ, in association with Guys Hospital.

The above have been selected from the very large number looked at by the authors, both for their content and attractive presentation.

USEFUL ADDRESSES

The Vegetarian Society (U.K.) Ltd, Parkdale, Dunham Road, Altrincham, Cheshire.

The Vegan Society, 47 Highlands Road, Leatherhead, Surrey.

6

Discussion of normal labour

It might be thought that two healthy young women who had both attended classes, had normal pelvic measurements, and babies of similar size presenting in a favourable position, would have similar labours, but we know that this is far from the truth. One will have a quick, straightforward labour with little pain, the other may have a much longer, more difficult labour and will react badly to the whole process. It is very hard to tell whether her attitude of mind is causing her apparently physical difficulties or vice versa.

It seems that even a first labour cannot be regarded as an isolated event in a woman's life. It is the culmination of her whole psycho-sexual development up to this time and her reactions to it will depend on her upbringing—particularly on her relationship with her mother—on her personality, and on her reactions to her bodily functions. If she has a wise mother who has spoken of birth as an exciting and worthwhile experience she will tend to expect the birth of her own child to follow this pattern. If her mother has encouraged her gradually to develop her independence she will approach any of the problems of birth or child-rearing as a mature woman, whatever her age. If, however, she has led a restricted life, continually dominated by a possessive mother, she will seek for a great deal of support from her antenatal teacher during pregnancy and her midwife or doctor during labour. Such women may behave well during the early phases of labour but blame the midwife, who often plays the role of substitute mother to them, and become angry and uncooperative if they meet with difficulties.

The personality of the woman and her relationship with her husband or partner also play a great part in her reactions to labour. The passive, feminine type of woman accepts the first stage of labour well but may become very disturbed by the turmoil of the second stage. The more active and aggressive types find the comparative inactivity of the first stage hard to tolerate and may become abusive to their husbands or midwives, but enjoy the effort of the second stage. A few very masculine women react in a different way, 'they consider childbirth an indignity imposed upon women by nature, an injustice that must be corrected' (Deutsch, 1947). Naturally they refuse to endure any pain or to participate in the delivery, they feel that it is the task of the obstetrician to make everything pass as quickly and painlessly as possible.

Niles Newton (1971), a well-known American psychiatrist who has worked in close collaboration with her obstetrician husband, believes that coitus and labour have many similarities and that the experience of the latter may be foretold by the girl's reaction to lovemaking.

When discussing a woman's expectations of birth, the influence of her peer group and of the mass media is not always appreciated. She may well demand an epidural anaesthetic because several of her friends have had one or announce her intention of nursing her baby in imitation of a famous personality.

Antenatal classes tend to attract those people who want to understand and play an active part in the experience of birth, but we shall have women of diverse upbringing and many different personality types. All those who work with pregnant women should be aware of the psychological as well as the physical factors which may influence their labours. We need to resist the temptation to play the amateur psychologist unless qualified to do so, or to expect that we shall change attitudes arising from deep-seated problems of upbringing or personality. We may, however, observe the effects of some of these during individual and group discussions and the interactions of class members with each other and with their husbands at fathers' evenings. Since it is our privilege to spend longer with these parents than any other member of the antenatal team we can sometimes spot and report reactions which we believe to be particularly unfavourable.

It is our job to relieve superficial fears arising from lack of knowledge about the processes and handling of labour, thus making the end of pregnancy happier, and to stress the satisfaction and joy in achievement of the birth of a child, reinforcing this aspect with any visual material that we use. By subtle manipulations of the group we can attempt to modify the aims of the extremists, trying to arouse interest in participation in some part of the process in those who just 'don't want to know', and to point out to those who picture themselves watching the birth of their babies in a state of undrugged bliss that there may be medical reason either for themselves or their babies why sedation or instrumental help may be necessary.

There will also be many middle-of-the-way people who are much less biased, who want to prepare themselves physically and mentally for the differing types of experience they may meet and to learn to help themselves and those who are looking after them to the best of their ability. By creating a realistic, purposeful atmosphere— hopeful but not rose-coloured—we hope to give confidence that they can cope with whatever their labour pattern turns out to be. In every case we must try to understand the goals that women and in some cases their husbands set for themselves, and beware that we do not replace these with what may turn out to be equally unrealistic ones of our own.

What does a woman want to know about labour?

1. What changes are going to take place in my body and how will I recognise their beginning?
2. What will they feel like and how may I react?
3. How will the staff look after me and what will they ask me to do?
4. How can I help myself?

As with the classes on pregnancy these points can be covered by talks, discussion and the practice of neuromuscular control.

METHOD OF PRESENTATION

Some teachers may wish to give a brief run-through of a normal labour and then break it down into stages considering each in some detail. Others prefer to divide the subject into three or four parts, discussing the physiology, psychology, management and self-help for each part, and so gradually building up a picture of the whole over two or three weeks. A few technical terms such as effacement, dilatation, expulsion and episiotomy, used always in the conjunction with the lay term or a simple explanation, help to dispel some of the professional mysticism. A series of simple diagrams on the board, such as those in Figure 4 in which the vaginal plug is removed with the sweep of a duster, the membranes rupture, dripping chalk drops down the board and the cervix dilates most realistically, make their point vividly and unemotionally. If one cannot draw, flannelgraphs or commercially produced pictures such as those from the Dickinson Belskie Birth Atlas or the Cow & Gate mothercraft charts are useful. We prefer the former since the baby looks much more attractive and the pictures of dilatation are larger. At the end of this chapter are some points which may be useful when 'talking through' the Birth

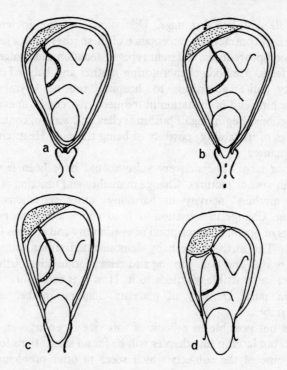

Fig. 4 Simple diagrams of birth: (a) early first stage: (b) late first stage; (c) second stage; (d) birth of the head.

Atlas. A pelvis, the models of the knitted uterus, and the baby and bowl or box described in Chapter 3, help in creating three-dimensional pictures. Each teacher, in her own way, needs to give her group something beyond the basic mechanics of the process and to inspire them to think about the wonderful design of their bodies and feel pride in being women able to give birth to a child.

Pre-labour stage. Possible signs: frequent contractions, weight loss, less activity from baby, spurt of energy in mother, wind in bowel sometimes with slight diarrhoea. Final arrangements and packing—keeping up morale.

Onset of labour. Final preparations, clothes and equipment needed. Variability of signs, excitement that waiting period is over, some apprehension, early contractions, what they do and what they may feel like—differences for multigravidae—what to do at home, when to go into hospital or call midwife.

Middle and late first stage. Dilatation, increase in length and strength of contractions, acceptance of these (they have a job to do), admission procedures, different types of sedation and analgesia, uses and effects. Methods of monitoring mother and baby. Transfer to delivery suite according to hospital routine. Symptoms of approaching end of dilatation in frequency, strength, unevenness of contractions. Beginning of pushing reflex and ways of controlling it. Feelings of irritability, possibly of being trapped. Heat, chill, shivering, nausea.

Second stage. The delivery suite should have been familiarised through visit or pictures. Change in quality and function of contractions, mothers' activity in harmony, other sensations akin to pushing. Change in sensation as head comes down on perineum, feelings of opening, description of episiotomy and reasons for it (see Ch. 6). The birth of the baby demonstrated either with doll and pelvis or doll and box, panting and relaxation to 'give birth', baby's appearance, possible reactions to it. How it is cared for.

Third stage. Delivery of placenta, making mother and baby comfortable.

It is not possible in a book of this size to enlarge on all these points, but later in this chapter will be found suggestions for dealing with some of the subjects which seem to offer problems to new teachers.

Physical signs and their management (topics 1 and 3)

Talks both on the physiology of labour and on its management may be given by the antenatal teacher providing she has a sufficiently close liaison with the delivery team; otherwise it is better that the conduct of labour should be discussed by the midwife or doctor who will be responsible for it. When it is not possible to make arrangements of this kind, then it is essential that the teacher should do everything she can to familiarise herself with current practice in the units where her students will be delivered, and if she is herself a midwife she must realise that some of these practices may be very different from her own. Difficulties sometimes arise in this country between local authority and other classes not closely associated with the maternity hospitals, and even in some instances inside the hospitals themselves, when several members of the staff have differing philosophies. One of the most striking things we have noticed about psychoprophylactic preparation in France is the complete integration between training and practice.

Sensations and reactions (topic 2)

If the group are all primigravidae discussion on sensations and emotions cannot be dealt with in the same way as during the 'pregnancy' classes, since labour is an unknown experience, but the group can be led to consider some of the factors in their lives which may influence their feelings about giving birth and to think about the solutions they may have found to other stressful situations they have had to deal with. If there are multigravidae in the group they will naturally talk about their previous experiences and even if these have not always been happy, they can usually be discussed in such a way as to offer a positive learning experience to the others. The women will undoubtedly be told horror stories by friends, relations and other expectant mothers awaiting their turn at the antenatal clinic; it would seem to be better to have some of these skeletons removed from their cupboards into the light of the classroom and looked at dispassionately. There are, however, a few multigravidae who need to unburden themselves without any thought for other people's feelings and these may benefit greatly from a private session with the teacher. If she is herself a mother, her talks on labour will be much more vivid, but she needs to beware of describing the whole process in terms of her own experiences. She may paint a more comprehensive picture by including anecdotes about other labours she has seen, reading letters from previous students, or inviting women from other groups who have had their babies to come back and talk about their experiences. Members of the group are usually very ready to ask questions or to join in the discussion, citing incidents told to them by friends and relations. Slides, films and tape recordings of labours can be very useful in triggering off discussion but they are highly emotive and need to be chosen and used with great care (see Ch. 3).

Pain in labour

When describing labour to parents perhaps one of the most controversial points is whether or not to use the word *pain*. The Russians believe that women are conditioned to expect labour to be painful by their mothers, their friends, the books they read and the films they see. They therefore interpret any unusual sensation in labour as pain and one of the aims of preparation is to decondition this 'labour equals pain' concept. On the other hand, what are the effects on a woman who has been led to expect only discomfort which she can control if she experiences sensations which to her are really painful? She may be frightened that something is going wrong with herself or her baby, guilty that she cannot fully control this unpleasant sensation and resentful towards her attendants.

We believe that most women do experience what they would describe as 'pain' at some time during labour and it is therefore better to use the word occasionally so that they may learn more about its manifestations, discuss them and come to terms with them. On the other hand, it seems unnecessary to reinforce the conditioning which certainly does exist by describing every contraction as 'a pain'.

In the book, *Pregnancy and Birth* Professor Frank Faulkner and Christopher Macy (1979) have written about pain sensations. They observe that we only have the word 'pain' for many sensations, ranging from pulsing or throbbing to burning or searing, and feel that Western languages have only crude terms to express internal experiences. They draw a parallel to the fact that Eskimos have sixteen words to describe snow, while we have only one—we have words for what is appropriate to express in our culture.

In Hebrew there is one word for pain, 'ka'ev', and another for the sensations of labour, 'tsirim', a near translation of which would be 'contractions'. So, Faulkner and Macy write, 'it makes perfectly good sense in Hebrew to enquire "are your tsirim giving you ka'ev?" ' We feel that, here, many teachers do as we do, and say 'at some point, the contractions will be painful', following this with examples of things to do to ease the pain, such as moving about, taking up different positions, and being massaged.

In the past, labour has sometimes been looked upon as a punishment for indulgence in sexual pleasure; indeed, even today, this concept is not quite dead when the mother is unmarried. It used to be something to be got through as quickly as possible and then forgotten, but now we try to present it as a challenging and exciting experience. It may involve pain, it will certainly involve patience and effort, but offers to most people the tremendous satisfaction of a job well done and the joy of bearing a living, healthy child.

Based on retrospective analysis of their patients, some psychiatrists believe that it is a disservice to women to deprive them of all birth sensations. Helene Deutsch (1946) says that, 'At bottom, despite her protests and pleas to be relieved of all pain, the woman wants to fight the birth pains largely with her own resources and is ready to accept a certain amount of pain for the source of the fullness of her experience'. We have certainly observed that women who have either been unconscious or very dazed at the time of birth seem to take longer to achieve a relationship with their babies. It is equally true that memories of severe pain or distress may mar the mother-child relationship. Perhaps the continued development of epidural analgesia, in which pain is relieved but sufficient sensation of the contractions remains for the women to take an active part in the second stage, is the answer, certainly during difficult labours.

Helping oneself in labour (topic 4)

This is concerned with building up the mother's morale during the talks and discussions so that she has a good idea of what to expect, including different kinds of support that will be offered by the labour unit staff, and is able to accept a number of possible patterns. By increasing her awareness and control of her own body, she feels confident that she can trust in it.

Each teacher will suggest specific methods of coping with labour based on her own experience and her adaptations of different theories. The Pavlovian proponents of psychoprophylaxis, in its initial form, have well-nigh disappeared, and verbal conditioning to produce a pattern of rigid breathing levels, as a distraction technique, is no longer thought to be good teaching. The firm base of the Dick-Read fear-tension-pain thesis is used by most teachers as their starting point, so a knowledge of what to expect in labour, and the ability to relax, remain essential. Since Michel Odent, and the 'active birth' movement, 'instinctive responses' to the sensation of labour have been strongly advocated. It is obviously too late to discover, in labour, that one's instinctive response is fright, so, however the teacher does it, it is essential to fix firmly in each woman's mind that her job during contractions is to 'let them work'. Relaxation and rhythmic breathing itself may not be 'instinctive'—indeed, most of us do not consider *how* we are breathing, and are unaware of our breathing becoming stressed when anxious. It is still valid, therefore, to practise breathing 'through' or 'over' a contraction—this can then, in labour, be a woman's conscious response. We feel that a woman must look forward to many strange sensations in labour, some of which will be painful, and that, given enough knowledge, relaxation, and conscious breathing control, she will feel more confident to meet these sensations. Each individual will react differently according to her upbringing, her personality, the length and course of her labour, and the way she is supported through it.

All we can do is to give her a number of tools, and encourage her to practise with them so that in labour she can use the ones which are appropriate to her individual position. Many women will want to lie down at the end of the first stage of labour, perhaps with the help of gas and oxygen, while more active women may feel more in control if they are standing, sitting or kneeling, perhaps meeting the rhythm of the contraction with the rhythm of pelvic rocking or swaying. Massage from a partner, either for its pain-relieving effects or simply as an expression of loving contact, may give one woman all the support she needs, while another may feel that the only way she can cope with the sensations is to have a rest from them by epidural analgesia. This is especially helpful in a long labour, when a woman's endeavours to remain in control have tired her. She may then need extra help in controlling and working with her body in the second stage, and should be assured that the midwives will be encouraging all her efforts.

When talking about 'helping oneself' it is essential that a teacher keeps up-to-date with methods used in the local maternity units. This is quite difficult, as the views of obstetricians and midwives are changing very rapidly at present. It appears, at times, that we are facing two diametrically opposed views of the management of labour—some hospitals encouraging maximum mobility while others are 'high technology' units using monitoring machinery throughout, which would mean that most of the labour would be inevitably spent lying down. In fact, this is not absolutely correct. Monitoring now is being used more selectively, with fifteen to twenty minute 'traces' taken of contractions and fetal heart rate when each woman is in established labour. If all is going well, the monitors can be removed to allow freedom of movement, and replaced at intervals for further checks. Although obstetricians decide overall policy in any unit, it is the midwife who can modify this policy to suit the needs of her patient. She observes, guides, suggests, and helps to maintain comfort. Two recent examples may illustrate this. The first was in a hospital where mobility was actively encouraged. When the midwife noticed that her patient looked more comfortable lying down, she helped her to relax on her side with lots of pillows, and taught her partner sacral massage to relieve a severe backache.

In the second hospital, monitoring was the rule, and the woman found that the two abdominal bands were uncomfortable and immobilising. The midwife fitted a scalp electrode to monitor the fetal heart, helped her patient to an armchair beside the bed, and checked the contractions occasionally with a gentle touch of her hand on the contracting abdomen.

Both these women found the experience rather different from their expectations, and much less stereotyped and rigid than they had been led to believe.

Perhaps, therefore, it is good for us, as teachers, to have to cope with diversity of methods and policies in the units we are teaching for. By getting all the class to practise coping with contractions in different positions—sitting, standing, squatting, kneeling and lying down—we are giving them a 'kitbag of tools', any of which can be used in their own individual circumstances. It is impossible to predict any labour—and every teacher should acknowledge that birth will be different with each experience, and each woman can choose the tools she herself needs. Most midwives have adapted now to the idea of letting a mother have as much choice as possible, and while some hospitals have gone as far as having a 'birthing chair' or 'borning bed' (see refs.) instead of traditional beds, in others there are wedges and pillows for sitting up, beds which can be lowered for the mothers to step in and out easily, and a comfortable chair by the side of the bed. The modern midwife is certainly not expecting a woman to 'take over' the management of her own labour, but is much more willing to be used as a resource of guidance and reassurance. She will help and reinforce the mother's own training and adapt to her wishes and efforts when possible. As one nursing officer said recently: 'We are here to be of service—to help the woman help herself. This is *her* labour, *her* experience'.

USEFUL EXPLANATIONS

Contractions—their job and how to cope with them

The subject might be introduced by asking the class how many of them have noticed that their tummies sometimes become very hard and may even point forwards slightly. This happens when the muscles of the womb have a practice session several times a day. The feeling can usually be differentiated from the baby's movements, since it is a slow tightening which may last a few seconds or even a few minutes before it slowly fades, whereas the baby makes rapid 'fish like' flips or sometimes gives really hard kicks. Members of the group who have felt these Braxton-Hicks contractions will describe them in different ways to help the others also to become aware of them. They will usually agree that the contractions are not painful unless they occur when the bladder is full but are by no means sensationless. One can then continue as follows.

'When labour begins, contractions are usually felt at fairly widely spaced intervals, may be quite weak and last only 30 to 45 seconds; as it progresses they gradually become longer, stronger and closer together. The early ones, and for some lucky people a large proportion of all the contractions, feel like those they have experienced during pregnancy, that is, a tightening, squeezing sensation of their tummies, for others they become uncomfortable and may become really painful. The sensation may be similar to the deep cramp-like ache of a period pain, it may be a low backache or occasionally an ache in the thighs.

'The sensation, whatever form it takes, is wave-like, it starts from nothing, increases to a peak, then dies away again. Except in unusual circumstances you will be quite comfortable during the intervals between contractions, and when these are long you may like to occupy yourself by moving around, reading, knitting, watching television, or talking to your husband. Later, as the contractions follow each other more closely, you will want to use the intervals to rest and gather your forces to cope with the next one. Some women do not have, or do not feel, any weak, widely spaced contractions—their labours start suddenly and their contractions come strongly at frequent intervals from the beginning; this is a common pattern if labour is started by the doctor (see inductions, Ch. 7).

'During labour the muscles of the womb, or uterus, have the power to contract and shorten, then to relax but remain in the shortened position. This results, first of all, in the gradual thinning out of the thick fleshy area round the cervix or neck of the womb and then in its gradual opening, and goes on until the cervix is wide enough open to allow the baby to pass through into the birth canal. This point is known as the end of the first part or first stage of labour.' (Demonstrate with diagrams, the hands, knitted uterus or offer the simile of pulling a polo-necked jersey over the head.) 'When you have had one baby the cervix does not become thick again so that it begins to open soon after contractions start and the first stage of labour is usually shorter. During the second stage of labour, the upper part of the uterus pushes down on to the baby, gradually pressing it along the birth canal and out into the world. These contractions may be quite painless but feel as if one has a tremendous piston inside one's body which makes one want to hold one's breath and go with it. Some people describe the sensation as similar to being constipated, getting half way through a motion and feeling that one *must* finish it, others as being an uncontrollable force like a hiccup, except that instead of something in one's body flipping up, it is a more sustained downward pressure that one feels.'

Thus we hope to establish contractions as a purposeful activity of the body, not as some useless disorder. In other circumstances, pain is feared and resisted as an indication of something wrong; here we can associated it with the progress of the baby along the birth canal, until it is hoped that a woman can say, 'Yes, I feel pain but this means progress and the contraction is the important thing, I must let it work'. It must be made clear that every woman has her own pattern and this may well be different for different babies.

Coping with first stage contractions. If you have learned the Mitchell method of relaxation try to think of your body opening up instead of being held in the typical flexed position with body, knees and elbows bent and shoulders raised. If you have learned other methods of relaxation try to picture yourself coming to meet the contraction and accepting it, not withdrawing from it and fighting against it, so that your body remains in harmony with your uterus. There are times, particularly towards the end of the first stage of labour, when you just cannot relax; don't worry, do your best and at least make sure you relax in between contractions. It is at this difficult stage that changing positions, with rhythmic movement such as gentle pelvic rocking, can be of great help during contractions (see Figs. 5, 6, 7).

'In the second stage of labour your behaviour will be quite different, you will be encouraged to cooperate with your contractions by using other muscles to augment the activity of your uterus so that your baby can move smoothly along the birth canal.

Pain relief in labour

As with all other aspects of the management of labour, it is important that the antenatal teacher should be in close touch with the methods in current use in her labour wards and should fit her remarks to these.

Common drugs

The three commonest means of pain relief in labour are epidural analgesia, pethidine, and nitrous oxide.

(It should be noted that anything which induces calm and tranquility also causes the production of endorphines—natural morphine

feeling that one «and hush it» makes an uncontrollable force
like a hiccup, except that instead of moving in one's body flipping
up, it is a more sustained downward force that one feels.'

'Thus we hope to create ... the purposeful activity of
the body, not as some ... in difficult circumstances, pain
is feared and resisted ... on in the time wrong; here we
can associated it with ... of the ... along the birth canal.
Until it is hoped that ... to say to ..., I feel pain but this
means progress ...... More important thing, I must
let it work. It ... makes clear ... every woman has her own
pattern and his ... well be different for different babies.'

Coping and progress can ... By. If you have lost not the Mitchell
method of relaxing ... and ... our body opening up instead
of being held in ... typical flat position, with, body, knees and
elbows bent and shoulders raised. If you have learned other methods
of relaxation try ... the structure you get control to meet the contraction
and accepting it, and withdraw ... from it and fighting against it, so
that your body remains in harmony with your uterus. There are
times, particularly towards the end of the first stage of labour, when
you just cannot relax; don't worry, you will be best and at least make
sure you relax in between contractions. It is at this difficult stage
that changing positions, with rhythmic movement such as gentle
pelvic rocking, can be of great help during contractions (see Figs 5, 6,
7).

In the second stage of labour your behaviour will be quite different: you will be encouraged to cooperate with your contractions.
By your further muscles to augment the activity of your uterus so that
your baby can move smoothly along the birth canal.

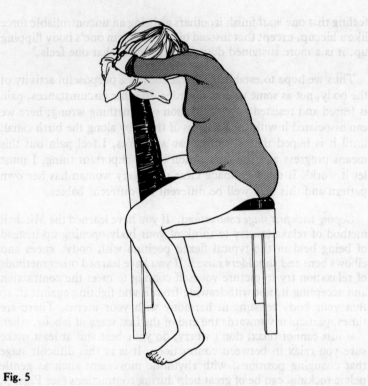

Fig. 5

Emergencies ...

As with ... at all ... our of labour, it is important that the ... ... close touch with the
mother ... ... she should in her remains aware.

General care

The first comment in this connected in labour analgesia epidural
analgesia, pethidine, and nitrous oxide ...
Here, should be noted that anything which reduces pain and tranquility increases the prospect of ... — natural means.

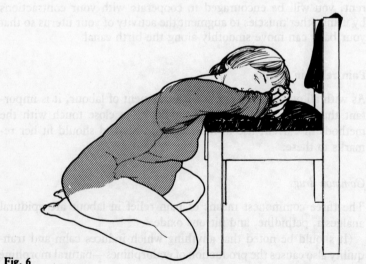

Fig. 6

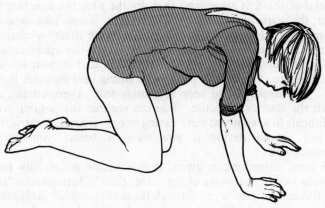

Fig. 7

like substances in the bloodstream. Endorphines have been found to go up at the end of pregnancy, and people who respond well to placebos have been found to make more endorphines naturally.)

Epidural analgesia. 'This is available in most hospitals today, as more and more anaesthetists are skilled in the technique. It is often used simply because you wish to have it, but it may be advised strongly by the medical staff, perhaps in a long or difficult labour, or if your blood pressure goes up.

Although mothers having first babies often use it at the end of the first stage, or before this if the labour is long and tiring, many mothers having normal labours seem to be deciding not to have epidural analgesia. It is certainly not used often in subsequent labours, by the mother's choice. The reason may be that many hospitals are advising women to arrive in hospital later, making themselves comfortable at home for as long as possible, and are teaching them, both when at home and in hospital, to move about more freely, using different positions for ease, and so the time spent lying in bed is much less. The midwives also are encouraging women to accept and 'go with' their contractions, and are encouraging husbands to provide more physical support, such as massage, as well as emotional comfort.

In fact you may find, if you go to hospital for your second baby, that the very midwives who were encouraging you to have an epidural injection will now be encouraging you to accept the contractions, and let them work, and later in the first stage offering gas and oxygen instead of the epidural injection. Sometimes, even if you ask for the epidural, you will be told that you have managed to reach the end of the first stage, and that, by the time the injection took effect, the worst bit of labour would be over. It does take some time to work properly and have its full pain-relieving effect—perhaps ten minutes after the actual insertion of the thread-like epidural tube.'

How is it done? 'You are usually asked to curl on your left side, with knees to chin, or may possibly be sitting bent forward. In both cases, it is important to keep absolutely still.' Demonstrate, after which the class can practise. 'You can see that the position would be difficult to keep if you were having strong, frequent contractions, so you should decide if you want it before you are too uncomfortable.

'A local anaesthetic is given, then a needle is carefully put in between two of the bones of the spine, there' (demonstrate) 'and a tiny thread-like tube is put through the needle and left in. If you get a contraction while this is being done, the anaesthetist will stop and wait for it to pass, so that you can keep still. The needle is taken out by being withdrawn up the tube, a filter is fixed to the end of the tube, and it is strapped to your right shoulder. Neither the needle nor the tube go into the spinal cord, just near it, inside the bony canal. An anaesthetic solution can then be put into the tube when necessary. If you are doubtful about whether you want it or not, a "cold" epidural can be performed in early labour. This means that everything is ready for when you want to have the anaesthetic.

'A "cold" epidural means that everything is in place, but only enough anaesthetic is used to be sure it is fitting properly, and no more until you wish it.' (With a cooperative maternity hospital 'team', a teacher may be given an epidural tube and filter to show to her classes.)

What will it feel like? 'A tiny prick for the local anaesthetic, then a dull pressure, and some people say a cold feeling when the proper anaesthetic goes in. Occasionally, there is a slight electric shock feeling down one leg. Then a numbed sensation in a few minutes— it is usually from waist to thighs, and sometimes your legs feel heavy. The numbing could be from waist to pelvic floor, so that the legs feel normal.' Here, people returning to talk about their labours, multigravidae who have had epidurals, or letters mentioning the sensations are useful. 'Each injection starts to wear off after two hours or less, and feeling begins to return. You are asked to tell the nurse before the sensation becomes pain, so that the "topping up" of anaesthetic is done quickly. However, you may have to manage one or two strong contractions before the next injection works. You can do this by concentrating on your relaxation and breathing techniques. More anaesthetic is then put through the tube, and the numbing sensation is as before. In some hospitals, the numbness is allowed to fade off in the second stage, and the pushing sensation is strong. In other hospitals, injections will be given right into the second stage, if the numbness fades. In this case, it is necessary to have taught yourself to push, and to be able to push accurately even when there is no sensation. The midwife will tell you when to push, and sometimes directs the push by pressing her hand on the perineum.

'Because of a natural fall in blood pressure with epidurals, it is better to lie on either side than to lie flat. Lying on your back makes the blood pressure fall more, and you would feel very dizzy. Sitting up can be comfortable if you don't feel dizzy when you do so.'

What effects will it have? When the epidural works well, the first stage will be painless and need no concentration nor effort. Your legs may feel very heavy, and you will need assistance to change your position. You will, of course, have to stay in bed. A 'drip' is always put into a vein (usually at your wrist) at the same time as the epidural procedure is performed. This gives you a solution of saline and glucose, which keeps you well nourished, but also can be used to insert other drugs quickly and easily, if needed. Sometimes, the blood pressure drops too low after an epidural, and drugs in the 'drip' control this and normalise the pressure.

The contractions will be monitored, either by a band round your abdomen or by a pressure gauge inserted into the uterus, and the baby's heartbeat is also monitored, either by an abdominal band or by a fetal electrode (see p. 156). As the contractions are painless, the midwives have to be able to see their strength, and how they are affecting the baby.

It may be difficult to empty your bladder because you feel so numb. If this happens, the midwife will empty the bladder by using a catheter (a small rubber tube) which of course you will not feel.

You may think that your labour has been 'taken over' and to some extent mechanised, but in a long or difficult labour this can be a great relief, and you will have the knowledge that you can have a rest, after, perhaps, coping with contractions for a considerable time.

After-effects. 'Usually none. Your legs may feel a little weak for a while, and very occasionally, headaches or backaches have been reported.'

Pethidine

How is it done? 'By injection, usually into the buttock, occasionally the leg, if the contractions are becoming too painful for you to control by your learned techniques, and if you wish it.'

What will it feel like? 'The doctor or midwife will have carefully balanced the dose, taking into account your body weight and also your normal reaction to drugs. This should mean that the pethidine makes you much more relaxed, less sensitive and life is seen through a rosy haze. You should still be able to control your breathing and muscular activity, with the contractions feeling much more comfortable. However, as the pethidine usually allows complete relaxation between contractions, you may doze, and feel that the contractions are coming nearer together than they were before. The injection takes about 10 minutes to work and wears off gradually over the next two to three hours. You will probably be asked to lie on your side after the injection, and not be allowed up to go to the lavatory, in case you are dizzy. The midwives will give you regular bedpans—it is still important to have an empty bladder.

'Pethidine can be mixed with other drugs, which relieve tension due to anxiety as well as pain, or have the effect of leaving little memory of labour. It is better, however, if pethidine is not given too close to the baby's birth—it enters the baby too, and can be traced in the body for eight days. For this reason, he is given an injection as an antidote to the pethidine at birth, usually if the pethidine has been given within six to eight hours of the delivery.'

What good/harm can it do? 'A mother is much more relaxed and able to cope with labour after pethidine. There are no after-effects. The baby is protected from after-effects by his injection, otherwise he may be sleepy or reluctant to suck.'

A new method for administering pethidine

An apparatus has recently been developed in Cardiff (Philipp, 1978) by which a mother can give herself as much (up to the limit set by her doctor) or as little pethidine as she feels she needs. To do this all she has to do is to press a button which activates the plunger of a syringe into a drip tranfusion that is placed in her arm. This is especially applicable if she already has a drip in place to speed up the labour, or to give glucose. She has to press the button twice to ensure that she does not administer a dose unintentionally. If she does not find that her pain is relieved adequately she can press the button a third and fourth time but then cannot press it again until a sufficient interval has passed for it to be safe for her to give herself another dose of pethidine.

Nitrous oxide. A midwife can show the Entonox machine to the group and let them try it out either in class or at the hospital where they are booked for confinement, or, failing this, they can see pictures of the apparatus in use. During a labour rehearsal the two hands can be cupped over the nose and mouth to simulate the mask so that the class can practise breathing deeply into it as soon as they imagine that a contraction is starting. The time lag of three to four breaths between starting to breathe the gas and its taking effect should be stressed, also the fact that it is under the mother's control and is harmless, making it safe to use right up to the time of the baby's birth.

A newer kind of pain relief—TENS (transcutaneous electro-nerve stimulation)

This is now being tried in several hospitals, but its use in labour is experimental as yet. Physiotherapists have used it successfully in sports injuries, rheumatoid arthritis and low back pain. Four pads are attached to the woman's back, and when she presses the control, a very small pulsed electric current passes through electrodes in the pads.

Hammersmith hospital has reported 'considerable pain relief' in eight out of ten of the patients using this machine. It is said to block pain signals at the 'pain gate' levels of the nervous system (see refs.).

The end of the first stage of labour

This is always difficult to describe since one is trying to make it sound tough without being too frightening. Here is one way of handling it.

'Some women seem to pass quite smoothly from the first to the second stage of labour: they begin to want to push, are encouraged to do so and the baby moves down the birth canal and out into the world. Others have a difficult time during this "transition" phase. You may be hopeful that the second stage is approaching when you notice a marked increase in the length and strength of contractions. If the bag of waters has not broken it may do so now, or be broken by the midwife; some leaking of watery fluid or spotting of blood is common. Sometimes contractions become uneven: you may have a big one then a small one or one that works up to its peak, begins to die away again, then just as you think you have coped with it, it comes back and hits you again. Some people describe this phase of labour as rather like trying to swim in a rough sea, you feel a bit battered but if you swim with the waves you emerge triumphantly into the calmer waters of the second stage.

'Other signs are a feeling of pressure on the tip of the tail bone at the height of contractions or a feeling of fullness in the bowel which makes you think you want to go to the lavatory but is in fact the pressure of your baby's head. You may find yourself burning hot, or shivering as if cold, making queer rumblings in your tummy or even occasionally feeling sick. Some women, who do not know much about labour, only really face up to the fact that they are going to have to go through with it at this stage and consequently feel trapped. You may hear somebody calling out that she doesn't want to have a baby today, and even you may find yourself getting rather short-tempered with the midwife or shouting at your husband.

'The best sign of all is the beginning of the pushing feeling, which was described when we were talking about contractions. This may mean that the neck of your womb is wide open and you will be told to go ahead and push, or you may not be quite ready yet. Sometimes the pushing feeling starts before the front rim of the cervix is completely drawn up, so that if you pushed too soon you would be trying to push your baby through a door that is not quite wide enough.' (Demonstrate with the clenched fist of one hand, trying to pass it through a space made by the index finger and thumb of the other hand.) 'You will therefore be asked not to push and may handle these contractions either with broken rhythm breathing' (demonstrate blowing breathing—see later) 'or by using the gas and oxygen mask with deep sharp breaths. Other women feel that they need more mental or physical activity to counteract these very strong contractions. You may help yourself by tapping the rhythm of your breathing; by counting up to the peak of the contraction, knowing that when you have reached a certain number the pain will begin to go; or by mouthing and tapping a tune. Also, remember that a change of position, massage, or movement, such as pelvic rocking, may bring relief. Even a good swear or a groan can relieve a lot of tension but do remember that a lot of noise will depress the other patients and annoy the staff. Between contractions the midwife may ask if the first stage ache of the contraction has become more of a pushing feeling. She will watch your perineum for signs of bulging, and may examine you vaginally to be sure that the cervix has been pulled up completely.

'At last she confirms that you can start to push.'

The second stage and the birth of the baby

'Now "labour" is indeed a true word. We shall be practising in detail the positions and breathing for this, and it can be a satisfying and exciting time, of sheer effort during contractions and rest between them. The midwives will be tremendously encouraging. Some women consider this to be bullying, but if you can imagine your helper as cheer leaders, or crowds encouraging an athlete, you will realise that they, by becoming involved in this emotional experience themselves, are helping you to overcome your tiredness and make the most of each contraction. The rectal sensation changes to a vaginal sensation as the baby moves further through the vagina, and soon in a contraction you will be able to feel the head moving down, and slipping back a little as the contraction ceases. This "two steps down and one back" action helps the vagina to stretch more easily. Remember it is very elastic, and the baby's head, which is quite soft and only measures about 9.5 cm or (3.75 inches) across, can stretch this elastic vagina bit by bit with each contraction, providing that you know how to work effectively and are prepared to "go with" the contraction and not hold back, which would cause tension and pain.

'Soon the midwife is telling you the colour of the baby's hair, and showing with her fingers' (demonstrate) 'how much of the head she can see.' Teachers should again be fully aware of local conditions— some hospitals will use a routine local anaesthetic at this point, whether an episiotomy (see Ch. 7) is performed or not.

'She will ask you to listen to her carefully, and issue orders to "push a little" then "relax and pant". Again we shall be practising this in class, and you will get the feeling, with practice at home, of real pelvic floor relaxation, so that the vagina can stretch without resistance. As you pant the head is born and a few seconds or perhaps minutes later the shoulders slip out, followed by the warm soft slippery body. You see the baby being held up which gives you a chance for a quick look at him, then he will be put at the bottom of the bed, more or less out of view, while the cord is cut and the ends tied. We'll call him male for convenience, but of course one of the thrilling moments is when you see whether you have a boy or a girl. He may need a tube put into his throat, to clear out any mucus or fluid he may have swallowed. A suction machine is usually used with the tube and you will hear its noise, then the baby crying vigorously, although of course some babies will cry immediately they are born. His breathing, pulse rate, limb movements, cry, and objections to being handled are all checked, and then he is wrapped warmly. He gets two points for perfect performance in each of these tests, so could get a total of 10 points. This is called the Apgar score as it was suggested by a Dr Apgar. Most babies will be below 10 at first, so may be given a little oxygen to revive them. Birth, after all, is tiring for the baby too. He is put in a warmed cot with his head down to drain any more fluid from his mouth and left to rest and recover. After four or five minutes his Apgar score is usually nine or 10 and he can be put into your arms.

'During those few minutes another midwife is busy with you. An injection will have been given in your thigh muscle after the birth of the head to cause a strong contraction, which you won't feel at all. The midwife rests her hand lightly on your abdomen and when she can tell by the contraction and the position of the uterus that the afterbirth or placenta has been squeezed out into the vagina, she gently levers the cord and the placenta slips out, feeling like a soft sponge. She put a pad between your legs and may ask you to put your legs straight down and cross your ankles. By the time you have been covered warmly and your pillows made comfortable the baby is ready to be cuddled'.

'Leboyer' deliveries ('Pour une naissance sans violence')

After watching many deliveries, Dr Leboyer of Paris questioned why babies, being freed from a constricted place, always seemed to cry and then sob when they were born. He stated that technically a newborn infant is hypersensitive through the skin, the eyes and the ears, and that birth was an assault on all these. He described the baby being handled insensitively, and bombarded with the lights and clatter of a busy labour ward. The cord was cut early and he believed that this caused sudden deep breathing, sucking air for the first time through the delicate respiratory tract, and creating pain.

In his Paris clinic, he instituted a system of peace, quiet and gentle loving stroking by the mother, immediately after birth. The room was half dark, and most of the noise was of the baby's first murmurings, and gentle breathing.

He was placed on his mother's naked abdomen, where, with skin to skin contact, she could easily hold him and stroke him. The father was also encouraged to stroke the baby gently. The cord was not cut early, as Dr Leboyer believed the baby received vital oxygen through the pulsating cord.

Then the baby was placed into a deep warm bath, returning as near as possible to his familiar environment. He was not washed, but just held lightly and allowed to regain his sense of weightlessness.

A film made of his techniques (see p. 236) shows the baby, with eyes open, observing the world with wonder and interest.

Since the publication of his techniques, many hospitals at least partly follow his example. There is more quietness after the safe delivery of the baby, gentle touching, and the mother is given him almost immediately to stroke and fondle, with skin to skin contact. The usual practice here is to put a blanket over mother and baby together, to preserve the baby's body heat.

There have been some criticisms of the method—some hospitals insist on bright lighting until mother and baby are seen to be doing well.

Others maintain that cutting the cord late may cause blood to pass back from baby to placenta, especially with early sepration of the placenta by the injection of syntocinon.

When Dr Leboyer was asked the essentials of his techniques, he replied 'Quiet, peacefulness, closeness'. This is now what many hospitals are achieving.

NEUROMUSCULAR CONTROL IN LABOUR

Relaxation

A first approach to the teaching of muscular relaxation by the contrast method has already been described in the chapter on pregnancy. However, it soon becomes obvious that a greater awareness of tension and degree of its control is necessary to cope with labour than simply learning to relax in comfortable conditions surrounded by known faces. Although the kind of relaxation practice in which the women are left to doze while the teacher goes away to make a cup of tea makes a restful interlude in their day, we do not believe that it is an adequate preparation for dealing with the challenge of labour or other difficult life situations. To do this it is necessary to accustom them gradually to relax in various conditions of stress. The following exercises can conveniently be practised in pairs, the mothers being encouraged to choose a different partner at each class so that they all get to know and help each other and to learn more about their bodies. Having seen that half the class are lying comfortably supported by as many pillows as needed and the other half are sitting or kneeling beside their partner, the teacher can demonstrate on one woman whose relaxation she knows is fairly good and who will not be embarrassed.

Relaxation when moved. Ask her to tighten her right arm and to note the sensations coming from her muscles while you feel them hardening under your hands, and then ask her to relax her arm so that both of you can feel the difference. Hold her hand just above the wrist, lift it and see whether her hand hangs limply off the end of her arm. Bend and stretch her elbow and see if the arm feels boneless (like a marionette with loose strings). Take hold of two fingers and pull the arm firmly towards you, lifting it a couple of inches off the floor and see whether it can be swung smoothly and heavily from the socket of the shoulder joint or whether, as often happens, at the beginning of practice she forgets to relax and holds up her own arm. Repeat the same technique by checking movements of the hip, knee and head Ask the rest of the class to try out these exercises and then to change with their partners.

The control necessary to achieve this type of relaxation is not the same as that used in labour, since contractions of the uterus are involuntary and the limbs are under voluntary control, but the exercise can give women a useful insight into the amount of concentration that is required, providing the reasons for it are clearly explained. A further and more meaningful progression can be achieved by arranging the women in a semi-upright sitting position, with bent knees, and asking them to hold their breaths, tighten their arms and allow their legs to relax and fall outwards without letting the breath go at the same time. This gives practice for pushing in the second stage.

Relaxation during discomfort. Ask one woman to place both hands on the inside of her partner's thigh and squeeze, gradually increasing her pressure until it becomes quite unpleasant. After a few minutes' pause, she repeats this, trying to apply the same amount of pressure, but this time the partner tries to minimise the sensation by deliberately relaxing towards the pressure and concentrating on slow deep breathing.

Nearly all teachers of relaxation for childbirth believe that this should be valuable in many stressful situations, not just in labour. To be meaningful, the teaching should first of all be associated with tensions or threats in everyday life.

Sheila Harrison has given us the following description of a piece of role-playing she uses at the beginning of a series of classes which she claims is highly successful in making a group aware of the effects of stress. She chooses a man or woman who looks interested, and requesting their help, sits them down in a chair with the rest of the class grouped closely around them. She suggests that the group should for example, pretend the model is waiting in the office for the results of a driving test. Mrs Harrison asks the group if the model looks the part and usually receives the answer 'No, he doesn't look anxious enough' 'Could you tell just by looking at him?' 'Yes'. 'All right, if that is so, give him instructions so that he looks tense; let's start with his shoulders, what would he do with them?' Somebody will say 'He would hunch them'. Moving down to his arms she is told of various signs of tension, such as: 'His elbows would be nipped in to his sides and his fists clenched. He would be sitting on the edge of his chair and leaning forward. His legs would be twisted together perhaps with one foot tapping; his jaw would be clenched and he would be frowning.'

So, after a while Mrs Harrison finds that the group has put the model into a position of tension; this is like the common flexion tension pattern of the 'fight, flight' reflex as described by Laura Mitchell. Occasionally when faced with a threat people take up an extensor tension pattern, particularly in labour. Frequently, the model himself complains that he is uncomfortable, and is getting tired; this makes it easy to point out that he is using a whole lot of unnecessary muscles. So we define tension as a bodily state when more muscles are working than are needed for the task in hand. Mrs Harrison then moves on to consider what else might be happening to her model. The group will tell her that his heart rate has gone up, his breathing is rather quick and shallow and has the emphasis on the intake of breath. To go on with the role play, when the examiner enters the room with the result the model gasps, then holds his breath. When he discovers that he has passed he lets out a sigh of relief, the tension disappears and the extra muscles stop working. Other role-play can be tried, such as sitting in a dentist's chair, watching a child cross a busy road, or going for an interview.

By now the members of the group will have a clear idea of the changes that tension can inflict on a person and can go on to learn how to relax or prevent tension from building up (see p. 33). They can discuss other situations when they might feel threatened, for example, waiting for an injection or a blood test, or for the women the anticipation of a vaginal examination or of a painful contraction in labour and wondering how they would deal with it.

Breathing in labour

It has sometimes been stated that deep breathing is necessary during contractions to maintain oxygenation, but Buxton (1966) has shown that hyperventilation with the resultant dangers of lowering the blood acidity is much more common than hypoventilation. He compared four groups of mothers, one untrained and three who had been taught various kinds of breathing for use during the first stage of labour. Hyperventilation was most marked in the untrained group but occurred also in the groups who had been taught to breathe very deeply and slowly and those who had learned very shallow rapid breathing. There was much less evidence of overbreathing in the fourth group, where less stress was laid on respiratory movements, and muscular relaxation was very carefully taught.

Various authors have advocated different types of respiration based on the use made of the diaphragm. Heardman used deep, slow breathing in which the diaphragm was encouraged to flatten and the abdominal wall to swell up to relieve pressure on the uterus as it tilted forward during contractions. Lamaze on the other hand, suggested very light shallow respirations in the upper chest to *minimise* movements of the diaphragm and so prevent any extra pressure on the fundus at the height of contractions.

Other teachers believe that respiratory control during the first stage of labour has a largely psychological value. Fairly deep slow breathing aids muscular relaxation and quiet concentration on the inflow and outflow of breath gives the mind a rhythmic focus of activity. We subscribe to this view but have found from experience and observation that somewhat shallower quicker breathing over the height of strong contractions seems to help many women. Whether this is due to the minimisation of diaphragmatic pressure or whether it is simply that a woman finds it helpful to vary her responses to a changing sensation and think of breathing 'over the top of the contraction' we do not know.

When the bearing down reflex is established, the maintenance of breathing control has a definite physiological basis as well as a psychological value, for it is the use of her diaphragm that determines whether a woman pushes well or not.

Breathing should always be as quiet and effortless as possible, and no commands other than to start or stop a particular kind of breathing should be given. Each woman is encouraged to find the speed and depth of breathing which is comfortable for her and then to maintain this when she is practising at home and later in labour. She will not always succeed but this activity in combination with carefully selected drugs does help to control the very rapid or very deep over-exaggerated breathing which one sometimes sees as a panic reaction in labour.

Breathing exercises should always be interspersed with other exercises and related to the type of contraction which they are designed to help. They may be introduced as follows:

Easy breathing. 'Whenever you want to relax, sigh out and let go completely, and now breathe just a little bit more slowly and deeply than usual, just enough to make you conscious of your breathing rhythm. Each time you breathe out try to feel a little bit more tension flowing out of your body. You will use this kind of breathing during early contractions'. (When the women have found the depth and speed that seems comfortable, they are each asked to time their respirations for a quarter of a minute; for a woman with a resting respiration of 16 to the minute, this slightly slower, deeper breathing comes out at about 12 to the minute.)

Lighter breathing. 'Put your hands on the top of your chests, just below your collar bones, and now breathe rather more lightly and quickly than before, feeling your chest rising and falling gently under your hands, rather like a pigeon ruffling its breast feathers. Don't forget that although you are breathing more gently then before, all the air that goes in must come out. You may prefer to let the air sigh in and out through half opened lips but make sure that you are breathing in your upper chest, not your throat, otherwise you will get a very dry mouth. You will probably find this kind of breathing helps you to cope with the peak of stronger contractions.' (Timing here results in a speed of 24 to 28 breaths per minute for most people, and mothers breathing more quickly than this should be encouraged to slow down and breathe a little more deeply.)

Demonstrate to the class as follows. Ask one woman to lie on her back, with her shoulders comfortably supported by pillows and knees bent. Having told her that you are going to give her a 'pretend' contraction, place your hands on her abdomen and begin a little gentle pressure—she breathes out and relaxes, then takes one or two breaths in her deep slow rhythm (in labour the number will depend on the speed with which the contraction builds up). Increase your pressure gradually over the next half minute, asking her to decrease her breathing depth as it becomes more comfortable to do so until she can picture the height of the contraction from your firm pressure and can 'breathe above it' with her shallow breathing. Release your pressure as the contraction dies away and she will hardly need to be reminded to slow and deepen her breathing again and to signal the end of the contraction with a big breath out. The class can then practise on each other.

Pushing breathing. 'Put three fingers on the soft spot above your baby and below your breast bone; now cough. Can you feel a ridge of muscle moving under your fingers? Try again, but instead of coughing, just make the ridge of muscle stand out again and feel that you have a piston' (or the plunger of an icing cylinder or anything similar which the girls will be familiar with) 'across your middle which is moving downwards.' (If anybody has any difficulty the teacher can demonstrate a strong push and let the mother feel the effort in her body, then try to copy this less vigorously.)

'This is a ridge of fat above the diaphragm, a big mushroom-shaped muscle which is attached to your ribs all the way round your body; above it are your heart and lungs and below it all the contents of your abdomen and pelvis including your uterus. When you breathe in deeply the centre of your diaphragm goes down as long as you hold your breath and keep your ribs *still*.' (Apart from pushing into the throat, the failure to fix or 'block' the ribs is the commonest reason for ineffective pushing, since movement of the rib cage gives the diaphragm an unstable origin to pull from.) 'In the second stage of labour, if you are asked to push, you wait for a contraction to start, take one or two deep breaths in and out while it builds up, then when you feel your uterus beginning to press down on your baby, you help it by holding your breath, making your diaphragm piston go down and at the same time tucking your head forward on to your chest to tighten your tummy muscles and increase the pressure. When you run out of breath you keep your position, breathe out, in again rather quickly, with head raised a little as if you were taking a quick gulp of air when swimming, and go on pushing steadily with the next breath until the contraction is over. Now rest back and relax completely.'

It is obviously not desirable that the women should strain during class but they do need to do just enough to be familiar with the correct sensations. The teacher can demonstrate either on herself or on members of the group, the different positions that they may be in. She may suggest that a woman should fix her eyes on a coloured tile or other point on the wall of the delivery room which she judges is about level with her vaginal opening and push towards this. Vague suggestions about 'pushing into your bottom' are not very helpful since the trained mother should be very well aware of where she is aiming. Stress should be laid on the necessity for relaxing the legs and pelvic floor and this will require some discussion on the possible sensations and emotions associated with the act of giving birth (see birth and the baby, later in this chapter). Above all, the class needs to be made aware of the power of uterine contractions at this time and the pleasure and sense of achievement that many mothers feel when they are working in harmony with them.

Breathing to prevent pushing. 'This may be used at the end of the first stage of labour if the cervix is not quite dilated or at the end of the second stage to allow the baby's head to be born slowly and smoothly. If your uterus is telling you to push and you are being asked not to go with it, you must do some sort of fairly deep breathing which will move the diaphragm up and down and stop it from fixing. Try a sharp blow out through a relaxed mouth, (demonstrate), 'feel as if you are blowing the pushing sensation away through your lips rather than allowing it to settle around your diaphragm. It may help you to concentrate and keep the rhythm if you tap on your thigh or count at the same time 1 : 2, 1 : 2. Alternatively your partner can put his hand on your upper chest and count for you; blow, in, blow, giving you a slight extra pressure on the outward blow. You can use this type of breathing and gain some benefit from inhaling gas and oxygen with the inspirations; it is more tiring but as it is usually used at the time your baby's head is being born, this is a matter of minutes only, so it does not matter. You may be told to "open your mouth and pant like a dog" but do remember to be a large St Bernard on a hot day, not a Pekinese in a hurry, because you *can* do very rapid shallow panting and push at the same time.'

LABOUR REHEARSAL

After discussing different aspects of labour and its management, we draw some of the common happenings together and offer the class at least two labour 'rehearsals': one of a straightforward spontaneous labour, the other envisaging some of the variations described in the next chapter (see especially the descriptions of inductions and epidural analgesia). Some teachers find the idea of presenting the women with a series of problems a somewhat macabre exercise, but we are thanked so frequently by past students for having given them opportunities to practise dealing with problems that actually happened to them, that we continue to do so. It certainly gives to the teacher a chance to check up on any information that has not been understood or remembered and gives the women the opportunity of imagining situations and finding the confidence to cope with them.

When painting a picture of labour, it is useful to 'talk through' a series of contractions at different stages including the mother's activities as well as the progress of the contraction; later, only a description of the contraction is given, leaving her to do what she thinks is appropriate. Diagrams for some of these have been included as a guide to inexperienced teachers who may later adapt them and change the words to fit their own experiences and understanding of their patients' normal life styles. Here is one possible outline:

'You felt very energetic yesterday and turned out several cupboards, took a little while to go to sleep because your back was aching but eventually had a good night's rest. You woke up about 5 a.m. to go to the loo and found a slight blood stain on your nightdress, got very excited about this and poked your husband but all the response you got was a sleepy grunt. You lay still for a bit trying to relax but turning over in your mind all the plans you had made— thinking about your suitcase, the baby clothes, your husband's supper if you had to go to hospital. Eventually having got it all sorted out and as nothing else seemed to be happening you went to sleep and did not wake again until the alarm went off at 7.30. After breakfast you had a couple of very loose motions and your tummy felt a bit uncomfortable, but gradually the discomfort began to come only periodically and you realised that your tummy was hardening each time, so guessed that these must be contractions.

'You had checked with your hospital during a visit and Sister had given you some instructions. She had probably said that unless your waters broke you could stay at home until your contractions were getting stronger and coming fairly regularly at eight to 10-minute intervals. Yours were still only vague and irregular, so you tidied up the flat and did odd jobs. You have remembered to empty your bladder every hour. Now maybe it is a couple of hours later and your contractions are getting longer and stronger and closer together. You are more comfortable now if you stay still as one begins, maybe resting back in a firm armchair, maybe standing or leaning forward on to a table or sideboard. Choose your own positions and let's imagine this type of early contraction starting now (Fig. 8).

'Now you decide it's time to go to hospital so your husband rings for the ambulance, you collect your belongings and off you go. You are put into a single room and your husband is asked to wait in the waiting room. You undress and get into bed and one of the midwives asks you to tell her what has been happening to you so far, and examines you, maybe just an external check of your baby's position and heart beat, possibly an internal examination. They say you are making good progress and decide to "prep" you in the way we have talked about.

'Now you have been to the loo and have been caught with a contraction in the corridor, what are you going to do about it? That's right, either lean forward against the wall, resting your head against your crossed arms or back against it with your hands in the hollow of your back. Breathe out and relax as the contraction begins, concentrate on your slightly slower, deeper breathing as it rises to its peak and fades, signal its end with a big breath out and continue on your way back to bed.

You may now be sitting in a chair, or in bed, with your husband sitting beside you. He may rub your back in the way we practised at the fathers' class or may try this if you have backache. You remember the pelvic rocking movement we learned in the early classes—it can also be helpful at this time but needs to be done very, very gently. Lie on your side, rock one way as you breathe in and the other way as you breathe out, experiment and see which seems best to you. Now let's use it through a contraction. It's starting now, breathe out and relax, in and rock, when you are ready you breathe

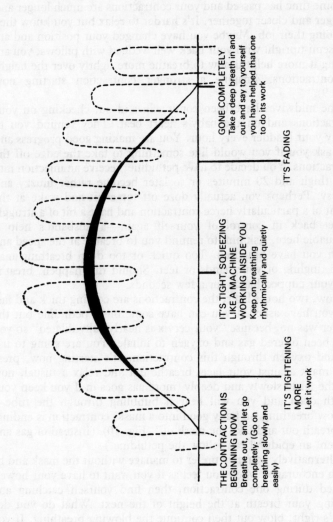

Fig. 8 Talking through a contraction. Early first stage (three-quarters of a minute to one minute). 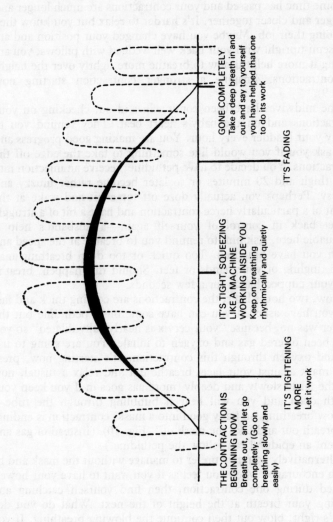 contraction; ------ breathing rhythm.

out again and rock the other way. Keep this up through the contraction and finish as usual with a big breath out. Throughout this stage it is a good idea to vary our position fairly frequently. Try sitting more upright or lying on your side, or moving about between contractions.

'Some time has passed and your contractions are much longer and stronger and closer together. It's harder to relax but you know they are doing their job. Maybe you have changed your position and are now semi-upright with your back well wedged with pillows; you are finding it more helpful now to breathe more lightly over the height of contractions. Imagine a stronger contraction starting now (Fig. 9).

'The midwives have been coming in and out checking on your contractions and on the baby's heart beat. They remind you to empty your bladder every hour. You are making good progress and they ask you if you would like something to take the edge off the contractions. You decide to have pethidine, receive an injection into your thigh and 20 minutes or so later become rather muzzy and drowsy. Perhaps you actually doze off for a bit and wake at the height of a particularly fierce contraction and have a bit of a struggle to get back in control of yourself again—a husband's help is invaluable here. Ask him to remind you to breathe at the speed and depth you have practised. Too quick or too deep breathing may cause tingling of your hands or feet. Should this happen, breathe into your cupped hands for a few seconds.

'Now, two hours later, the contractions are coming thick and fast and you have asked if you can have some more pethidine but the answer was no, because "your cervix is nearly fully dilated" so you have been offered gas and oxygen to inhale. You are going to use gas and oxygen through this contraction. It's starting now, press your mask against your face, breathe out and relax as usual, now breathe fairly slowly and deeply (more gas goes in if you keep your mouth open and you will hear it bubbling through the tube—shallow breathing isn't any good into a mask) contraction is ending, big breath out and take the mask off' (Fig. 10). (Instead of gas and oxygen, an epidural can follow the pethidine.)

'Alternatively you may prefer to manage without the mask and be much encouraged when you feel as if you want to have your bowels opened during one contraction, then find yourself catching and holding your breath at the height of the next. What do you do? That's right, blow out then continue the blowing breathing. If you are alone when the contraction is over, you ring your bell and ask a midwife to come and look at you. Perhaps they will say you are ready to push or perhaps you will have a sticky half hour in which you are being told not to push and you cope by fixing your eyes on

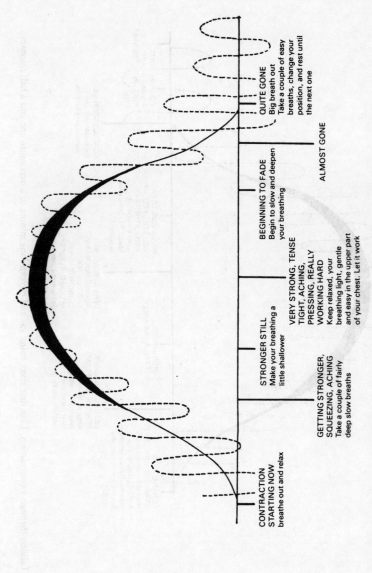

Fig. 9 Talking through a contraction. Late first stage (one minute to a maximum one and a half minutes).

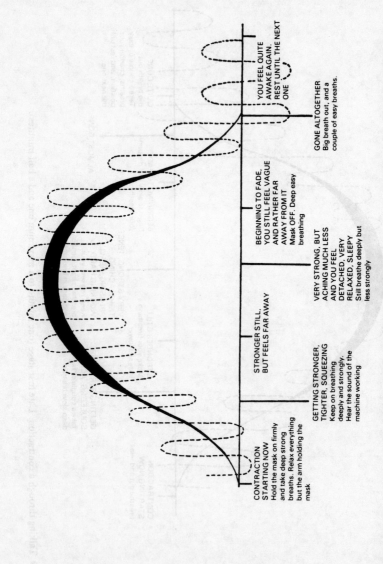

Fig. 10 Talking through a contraction. Late first stage using gas and oxygen (one minute to a maximum one and a half minutes).

your husband's face, continuing the blowing breathing, and tapping the rhythm against your thigh (Fig. 11).

'Your cervix is fully dilated now, and if not already in the delivery room, between contractions you will roll off your bed on to a stretcher and go along there. Here you are on a rather hard couch with a big light above you, surrounded by figures in masks and gowns; one of the midwives whom you can only recognise by her eyes, makes you comfortable, puts her hand on your tummy, says there is a contraction coming and you can try a little push this time. Everything you have heard about pushing goes straight out of your head but she reminds you (Fig. 12).

'The first few pushes don't go too well, then you get the hang of it. Perhaps your husband or the midwife can help by supporting your shoulders or helping you into a different position. Don't forget to relax completely in between pushes. Some women become very chatty at this time and will have a long conversation about whether they want a girl or boy or what they are going to call it, others just flop out and apparently go to sleep. You are beginning to feel tired, then suddenly revive when somebody says they can see your baby's head.

'You may now feel that the stretching sensation when pushing is distinctly uncomfortable. Some people do, and some actually say it feels extremely enjoyable. Remember that no two labours are alike, and even if you have six you'll find many differences. If you have had a local anaesthetic at this point the stretching feeling will be considerably diminished. If it's your second or third baby the stretching has already been done once and can be done easily and quickly again. Perhaps you might be just a bit apprehensive and think that it could be going to hurt soon. This will stop you relaxing the perineum fully and making the most of the contraction. It often helps to take two or three good breaths of the gas and oxygen, if you feel like this, at the very beginning of a contraction, then drop the mask and go into the pushing routine. This bit of extra help gives confidence to let you work well with your body.

'Now the baby is about to be born. The midwife asks you to do exactly as she says. Let's practise this contraction (Fig. 13).

'The vagina feels quite tense as the head slips out, even though you are consciously relaxing the whole perineum and your legs as you have practised. When asked to pant, remember that your mouth should fall slackly open. Some people, again in case it might hurt, like to have the gas and oxygen mask to pant into for these seconds. We could practise that too, relaxing the body except the one hand which holds the mask. You might not want to use it at all, and certainly very few people having second babies do, but just like to keep it by your hand in case you do.

'There is a sudden relief of pressure and gently the shoulders and

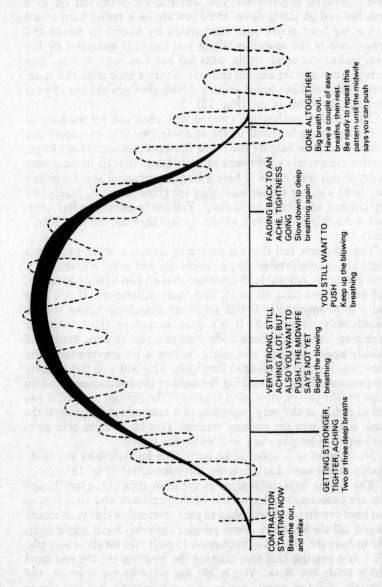

GONE ALTOGETHER
Big breath out.
Have a couple of easy
breaths, then rest.
Be ready to repeat this
pattern until the midwife
says you can push

**FADING BACK TO AN
ACHE, TIGHTNESS
GOING**
Slow down to deep
breathing again

**YOU STILL WANT TO
PUSH**
Keep up the blowing
breathing

**VERY STRONG, STILL
ACHING A LOT, BUT
ALSO YOU WANT TO
PUSH. THE MIDWIFE
SAYS NOT YET**
Begin the blowing
breathing

**GETTING STRONGER,
TIGHTER, ACHING**
Two or three deep breaths

**CONTRACTION
STARTING NOW**
Breathe out, and relax

Fig. 11 Talking through a contraction. Transition stage (one minute to one and a quarter minutes).

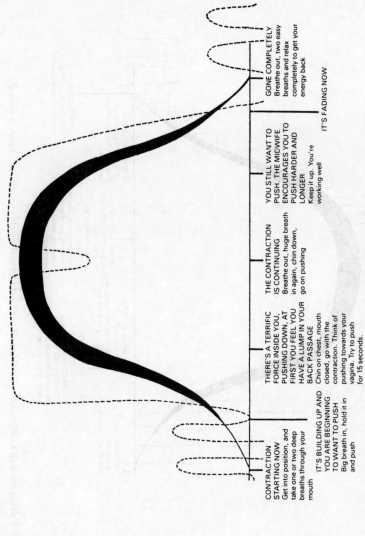

Fig. 12 Talking through a contraction. Second stage (approximately one minute).

CONTRACTION STARTING NOW
Get into position, and take one or two deep breaths through your mouth

IT'S BUILDING UP AND YOU ARE BEGINNING TO WANT TO PUSH
Big breath in, hold it in and push

THERE'S A TERRIFIC FORCE INSIDE YOU, PUSHING DOWN, AT FIRST YOU FEEL YOU HAVE A LUMP IN YOUR BACK PASSAGE
Chin on chest, mouth closed, go with the contraction. Think of pushing towards your vagina. Try to push for 15 seconds.

THE CONTRACTION IS CONTINUING
Breathe out, huge breath in again, chin down, go on pushing

YOU STILL WANT TO PUSH. THE MIDWIFE ENCOURAGES YOU TO PUSH HARDER AND LONGER
Keep it up. You're working well

IT'S FADING NOW

GONE COMPLETELY
Breathe out, two easy breaths and relax completely to get your energy back

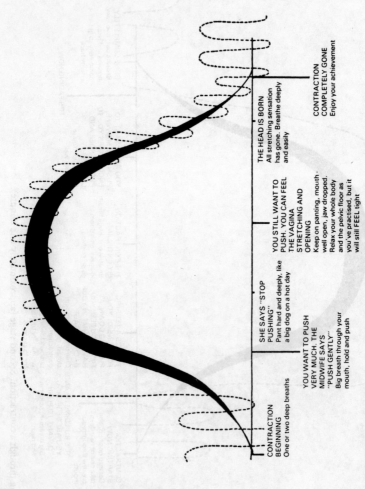

CONTRACTION BEGINNING
One or two deep breaths

YOU WANT TO PUSH VERY MUCH. THE MIDWIFE SAYS "PUSH GENTLY".
Big breath through your mouth, hold and push

SHE SAYS "STOP PUSHING"
Pant hard and deeply, like a big dog on a hot day

YOU STILL WANT TO PUSH. YOU CAN FEEL THE VAGINA STRETCHING AND OPENING
Keep on panting, mouth well open, jaw dropped. Relax your whole body and the pelvic floor as you've practised, but it will FEEL tight

THE HEAD IS BORN
All stretching sensation has gone. Breathe deeply and easily

CONTRACTION COMPLETELY GONE
Enjoy your achievement

Fig. 13 Talking through a contraction. The birth of the head (approximately one minute). *Listen to midwife.*

the rest of the body are slipping out. Look at your baby—he will probably look beautiful to you even though he is bluish, wet and sticky, perhaps a little bit bloody, and has a head shaped rather like an acorn.

'Your work is over, and you can rest with legs apart while one midwife takes care of the third stage, and another the baby. The placenta has arrived, you have a pad on, you are covered up and holding your baby, who by now has probably stopped crying and is lying peacefully.

'We can't try to tell you how you will feel at this minute. Most women say it is an indescribable feeling in any case. You will have to wait and see. You may feel tired and pleasantly happy, or exhilarated, you may feel instantly maternal, emotional and protective, or may at first view the baby with considerable detachment and be surprised that you should feel like this. Some mothers instantly feel overwhelming love, in others it has to grow over days or weeks. Accept your own feelings, hold the baby closely, and don't forget to let your husband have his share of holding him too.

'If you want to breast-feed, and your baby seems to be trying to suck, you might like to ask the midwife if you can put him to your breast for a minute or two. Many experts believe, as with most animals, a baby's sucking reflex is at its strongest just after birth if he is not too tired, and now midwives are often actively encouraging this early breast feeding. You and your baby will be helped to get to know each other, right from the first minutes after birth.'

DEMONSTRATING THE DICKINSON BELSKIE BIRTH ATLAS

This, like the Cow & Gate Mothercraft Charts, is designed so that it stands firmly without support, and the black-and-white photographs of the models are clearly and easily seen by a group of up to 15 people.

One could stand behind each picture and read the very good explanation of each model to the class. This, however, besides being dull and boring, would obscure the teacher, prevent her from observing class reaction, and hinder her from pointing to details. We normally sit on the floor by the side of the Atlas, with the class on mattresses or chairs as they please. A teacher on the same level, or lower, than her class has less of the didactic 'schoolmarm' image and this leads to a more relaxed group.

The explanations to each picture should, of course, be well learnt, then one's own words give spontaneity.

Here are a few points, put simply, that we have found worth mentioning:

Plate 1. Pelvis and uterus. Picture of pelvis demonstrated with, if possible, a model pelvis against teacher's body. The opening in the basin of the pelvic floor is described with its sling of muscles, and the model pelvis used to describe 'head engaged' and 'head fixed', etc. 'The growth of the uterus has taken place with no pain, even though everything else has got a bit squashed. In labour there is little pain from a uterine contraction itself; most of the pain or discomfort during the contraction is because the baby is being pressed on the muscles round the uterus as it comes lower with each contraction.

Plate 2. Female pelvic organs. One must emphasise that the woman is on her back—'legs here, tummy and breasts along here, and this the curve of the tail of the spine'. Always, at first, a simple word followed by the correct term—back passage or rectum, womb or uterus, front passage or urethra. 'It is obvious that all these organs have lots of room, but we shall see how everything becomes rather squashed by the womb later.'

Plate 3. Insemination, ovulation and meeting of sperm and ovum. 'This is vastly enlarged. The egg or ovum is as small as the head of a pin, so you can imagine how small the sperm are—but they are very much alive, and hundreds of them reach the egg, even though only one sperm enters. The bottom picture shows the fertilised egg becoming a cluster of cells within three days.'

Plate 4. Early weeks of development. (1) 'This is the day that your period should start, and here's an enlarged picture of the little ball of cells which is now firmly fixed to the wall of the womb. (2) Here you are two weeks overdue. This eight-times enlarged picture is beginning to look a little like a baby. (3) Three weeks overdue. Arms and legs growing and he has blue eyes. (4) Two and a half months pregnant. A real little baby, his heart is beating, fingers and toes forming, and he's almost filling the womb. The afterbirth or placenta is growing bigger and feeding the baby through the cord. He's moving a little, but not enough for you to feel him. (5) Three and a half months pregnant. He's got everything but fingernails, toenails and hair, and he's moving much more.' With the last two pictures it is very common for an argument to start in the class about the ethics of abortion—many women do not picture such a 'real' baby when abortion is discussed casually.

Plate 5. Four and a half months. The model pelvis is useful again here, against the teacher's body, to get the right perspective. 'At four and a half months pregnant he's kicking regularly and turning somersaults sometimes. He can get the cord twisted round him

during these "looping the loop" sessions, but this isn't important—
if it's round his neck at birth the midwife either clamps it with
forceps, then cuts it and unwinds it, or just loops it over his head.'
Usually somebody in class says that parents, grandparents, etc. have
warned about any pregnant woman putting her arms above her
head—'the cord goes round the baby's neck'—so this old wives' tale
can be refuted.

Plate 6. The function of the placenta. 'Just as a plant is fed from
its roots, through the stem to the leaves, you can see the afterbirth
as the roots, the umbilical cord as the stem, and the growing baby
being fed.' Here is an opportunity to mention diet and regular elim-
ination, and also that the mother's and baby's blood does not
actually mix, the placenta acting as a complicated sieve. It is as well
to be aware of what the placenta *does* pass to and from the baby, in
case one is asked if a baby can get chickenpox (it can) or tuberculosis
(it cannot) or to explain the Rhesus factor.

Plate 7. The baby at seven months. This is a delightful model which
the mothers relate to as their babies are about this stage (seven
months plus) and they want to know details of weight, length,
possibility of survival.

Plate 8. Before labour begins. Nine months, ready for labour. 'The
baby is lying sideways. As labour goes on he will turn until his head
faces to the back—if you look down to watch him being born you
will usually just see the back of his head. Note how closely the baby
will be pressing on the bladder—this must be kept as empty as possible. He'll have to squash the rectum a bit too and that's why you may
have a small enema, just to have that part of the back passage empty
to give him more space. Notice how thick the neck of the womb or
cervix is.' Pull up the page to show the cervix in the next picture
and compare the two. 'If you've been in labour at home for quite
a while, and when examined in hospital the midwife says the cervix
is only one finger dilated, ask her if it's thin, and then think what
a lot of work has already been done.' The dilatation of the cervix
can be demonstrated by one of the models described in Chapter 3,
or by the hands, using words which the midwife will use. One must
therefore find out whether she will talk of 'fingers dilated' or centi-
metres, and the class must be reassured that if she says 'four fingers
dilated' she is only using two fingers and seeing how far she can open
them.

Plate 9. Labour—cervix dilating. 'Notice how uncomfortable you
would be with a full bladder now, and it would also make labour
slower because the head would have less room. The baby has gone
deeper into the pelvis and is beginning to turn. He doesn't help
himself at all—he's pushed round by the contractions.'

Plate 9A. Labour—first stage. 'The cervix is half dilated. The bladder and back passage are both being flattened, especially during a contraction. In this case the waters haven't broken—you can see the membrane in front of the baby's head.'

Plate 10. Labour—second stage. 'The last bit of the cervix has opened and the womb and vagina make a continuous passage. The vagina stretches out just like one of those old-fashioned tightly pleated skirts, and goes back again to almost its normal size as soon as the baby is born. The membranes still haven't broken. At this point the midwife or doctor would break them (they may do this earlier) simply by a vaginal examination and pressing the bag during a contraction, when the bag bulges by the pressure of the shortening womb. The water flows out and feels warm. The baby's head is now changing shape. The bones are so soft they can do this easily, and there are even some points in the head, round the two soft spots, where the bones can overlap. The head's diameter is less than 10 cm (4 in) as it is being born—long and thin—but it gets back to normal in a very short time.' The class is often interested to be told that an experienced midwife can easily walk along a line of cots containing new babies and say 'that was a Caesarean section' because of his round head.

Plate 11. Labour—'crowning'of baby's head. 'The baby's head is almost completely turned to the back. The midwives can see part of it and are getting very excited as they encourage your pushing efforts. Just when you feel you could really push your hardest they will suddenly say, "Stop pushing and pant".'

Plate 12. Labour—second stage nearly completed. 'You are relaxing and panting, and the baby's head is coming out slowly, so that any tear you have can be as small as possible. The midwife's hands aren't shown, but she is guiding the head out.'

Plate 13. Birth. 'The top shoulder is born first and to manage this the baby is pushed by the next contraction into a sideways position again. The midwife waits for the head to turn (if it didn't the baby wouldn't be comfortable) and when it turns she knows the shoulder is ready to be born. She presses the head down a little, the top shoulder comes out, and the whole baby slides out smoothly, feeling warm and wet. He will be blue or mottled or bruised looking at first, but will get pink as he begins to cry. He may have a little blood on him, and almost always some grease as if he'd been coated with lard or Nivea cream. You will still think he looks beautiful!'

Plate 14. Third stage. 'The biggest contraction, but you don't feel it because there's no baby left inside to press on your surrounding muscles. The womb squashes down hard, the placenta can't change its shape so is pushed off the wall of the womb. The midwife helps it out by pulling the cord gently. Immediately the womb which had filled the whole page is as small as this. The midwife can feel it by pressing your abdomen—it feels like a cricket ball.'

Plate 15. Involution. (1) 'Five days after the birth—uterus still a little large. (2) Fourteen days afterwards—it has disappeared behind the pubic bone' (demonstrate on self) 'and everything is more or less back to normal. Pelvic floor exercises *must* be kept up at home so that the muscles which have become stretched become strong again.

Plate 16. Newborn baby. Describe the umbilical cord and what happens to it. Describe the dryness and sometimes cracking of the skin of the feet and hands, especially if the baby is overdue. It is possible that the regular movements of the baby's feet and hands inside the uterus rub off the protective grease and so the dryness occurs.

Plate 17. Twins. We tend to miss this out unless someone in the class is suspected of carrying twins, then we explain about the two layers of membrane and how identical twins share the outer layer.

REFERENCES

Buxton, R. St J. (1966) *Maternal Respiration in Labour.* Obstetric Association of Chartered Physiotherapists.
Deutsch, H. (1946) *The Psychology of Women.* London: Heinemann.
Leboyer, F. (1975) *Birth without Violence,* English edn. London: Wildwood House.
Macy, C., Faulkmer, F. (1979) *Pregnancy and Birth. Pleasures and Problems.* London: Harper and Row Ltd.
Newton, N. (1971) *Maternal Emotions,* 4th edn, p. 87. New York: Hoeber.
Phillip, E. (1978) *Childbirth,* p. 81. London: Fontana.

FOR FURTHER READING

Beels, C. (1978) *The Childbirth Book.* London: Turnstone Books.
Berezin, N. (1980) *The Gentle Birth Book.* London: John Murray. New York: Simon and Schuster.
Boyd, C., Sellers, L. (1982). *The British Way of Birth.* London: Pan Books.
Breen, D. (1975) *The Birth of a First Child.* London: Tavistock Publications.
Chertok, L. (1969) *Motherhood and Personality.* London: Tavistock Publications.
Dally, A. & Sweering, R. (1965) *A Child is Born.* London: Peter Owen.
Dunn, P. M. (1976) Obstetric delivery today. For better or worse? *The Lancet* 10 April.
Garrey, M., Govan, A., Hodge, C. & Callender, R. (1980) *Obstetrics Illustrated.* Edinburgh: Churchill Livingstone.
Gaskin, I. M. (1979) *Spiritual Midwifery.* Summertown, Tennessee: The Book Publishing Company.
Health Education Council *How a Baby is Born.* A very simple clearly illustrated leaflet suitable for those with poor English.
Huntingford, P. (1979) Obstetric practice—Whose baby? *Update* 15 June.
Kitzinger, S. (1982) *Birth over Thirty.* London: Sheldon Press.
Moir, D. (1982) *Pain Relief in Labour,* Edinburgh: Churchill Livingstone.
Myles, M. (1981) *Textbook for Midwives,* 9th edn. Edinburgh: Churchill Livingstone.

National Childbirth Trust (1972) *A Guide to Labour for Expectant Parents*, Leaflet No. 7.

National Childbirth Trust Book (1980) Loader, A. (ed.). London: Oxford University Press.

Perkins, E. R. (1980) *Education for Childbirth and Parenthood*. London: Croom Helm.

Prince, J. & Adams, M. (1978) *Minds, Mothers and Midwives*. Edinburgh: Churchill Livingstone.

Stirratt, G. (1981) *Obstetrics*. London: Grant McIntyre Ltd.

7

Variations of labour patterns

Some antenatal teachers with whom we have discussed the content of classes are strongly of the opinion that only 'normal' labour should be mentioned, as they feel it is creating fear and alarm to give details of abnormal labour patterns or obstetric procedures.

If, however, the three-part talk, practice, group discussion plan is followed, it is impossible, even if advisable which we do not believe, to avoid being asked questions of all kinds, many of which will refer to labour variations. We believe that these can and should be discussed, giving absolutely true and real explanations, but remembering that each woman will picture herself in the situation we are describing. Words should be chosen which are simple and undramatic, so as to leave an image which is neither frightening nor worrying. Long and technical descriptions should be avoided as they may not be properly understood.

In syllabus examples it will be seen that variations are planned to be discussed in one of the later classes. We have found, in fact, that most of the content of this talk will have been asked spontaneously in previous classes—and asked at the time when the questioner was really wanting to know, perhaps because of interest, but maybe because of sudden fear, and an explanation at that point is far more valid and remembered. This means that a teacher must be aware of points already covered in class, and a useful way of remembering is to make brief notes at the end of each session on questions answered. Indeed, this is essential if a teacher has several groups each week, at different points of the syllabus.

The talk on variations, therefore, is simply a reminder of explanations previously given, answering any questions which arise from this, and the addition of any topics which have not been asked in class.

The following topics should be covered at some stage during the course:

Inductions
A very short labour
A very long labour
Precipitate labour—what to do at home
Cessation or slowing of uterine contractions
Posterior positions
Breech positions
Fetal heart monitoring
Fetal blood sampling
Episiotomy, pudendal nerve block, local anaesthesia
Forceps delivery
Ventouse vacuum extraction
Caesarian section
Twins
Retained placenta
Differences in hospital bookings

In discussing these topics there are certain questions which frequently recur. Basically, whatever is to happen, a woman wishes to know:

Why is it happening?
With an obstetric procedure, how is it done?
What will it feel like? How can I help myself?
What good or harm will come to me or my child?

Even if a teacher does not wish to discuss any of the above topics as a routine in her class schedule it is wise to familiarise herself with all the subjects mentioned, and decide how she would reply to any question. She can, of course, admit that she does not know the answer, but if she promises to find out she must not fail to do so, or she loses the confidence of her class. (Again, a notebook is useful.)

USEFUL EXPLANATIONS

The following are brief notes on simple answers for teachers to consider when planning their own individual style of explanation.

We are starting with the most common variation, which is always mentioned in class—episiotomy, or 'what if I have to be cut?'

In recent years, there has been great argument about episiotomy. If one reads Robert Bradley's *Husband-Coached Childbirth* one is left with the opinion that it is an essential part of giving birth—indeed, that if it isn't done, not only will married life suffer, but a prolapse is more or less inevitable. This was the American view for years. Now read Sheila Kitzinger, and episiotomy, now that circumcision

is out of fashion, becomes the unkindest cut of all. Reality lies somewhere between these two extremes.

With the upright or semi-upright second stage, the episiotomy
rate has dropped. It appears that the baby's head is pushed round
the curve of the birth canal more smoothly, and steadily thins the
perineum as it descends. With less haste in the second stage, the
vagina has time to stretch, and all the muscles to 'give'. Certainly,
the statistics in some London hospitals have fallen from a 70 to 80
per cent episiotomy rate to perhaps 30 per cent for a first baby. This
still means perhaps a third of the class, but it does mean that we can
truthfully say it is *not* done routinely, and, with skilful midwifery,
is only done when the perineum has become so thin that it is obvious
that a tear cannot be avoided.

This has the advantage that the muscle which is cut has had time
to thin and stretch. Nobody today is going to cut through a thick
perineum unless there is an absolute need to do so, perhaps because
of a changing fetal heart pattern or because a forceps delivery is
necessary.

The cut in a thin perineum can be small, and has no need to be
'mutilating'. Again, there is controversy about the pain from a
healing stitched tear in comparison to the pain from episiotomy
healing. If there were no episiotomies in normal birth, there would
certainly be some third degree tears, and the pain of healing stitches
when part of the anus has been involved is infinitely worse than an
episiotomy. We can only refer readers to some views on the subject,
and invite you to form your own opinions, and present the truth,
or what you feel to be the truth, as you see it.

Here is one version.

Episiotomy

'This is a small cut, made in the muscle between the vagina and the
back passage—the perineum. We have been practising relaxation of
this bit of the pelvic floor, and in the second stage of labour some
of you will be able to push your babies out without tearing the
perineum at all. Others will have a small tear in the skin, needing
a few stitches.

As the head comes down, and round the curve of the birth canal,
the vagina stretches and widens, and the head rests on the perineum,
causing it to become thinner. If it becomes so thin that a tear seems
inevitable, then the midwife will use a local anaesthetic spray, or an
injection, then make a small cut, usually slightly sideways towards
the back passage.

You will not feel this, but she will tell you when she is going to do it. This is the time when both you and the midwife must trust each other—she must trust you to get the baby's head out with control, and you must trust her to make the cut only if it is really necessary. Talk to her about it beforehand, and be sure you both understand each other. If you really feel you would prefer a small tear to an episiotomy, say so. She will then tell you how things are going, and if the perineum is so tough that it is slowing the second stage, will help you to change positions and perhaps lean forwards to try to get the baby's head round the corner. If she knows your feelings, you must believe her if she eventually says that an episiotomy has to happen. You will both have tried your best.

At least, a straight cut is easier to sew up than a jagged tear. Stitching takes a long time—the doctor or midwife does it, with neat small stitches which will eventually dissolve. She will use a local anaesthetic, and you should be able to rest comfortably, holding your baby, while the stitching is done. If it starts getting painful, say so. More local anaesthetic can be used.

Stitches do hurt quite a bit, especially when all the local anaesthetic has worn off and the bruised muscles swell—which is usually the second day.

Warm baths feel lovely, and a little salt in the bath is, strangely, very pleasant. The swelling improves and healing is speeded up.

In a few days, the perineum should feel comfortable again, but until it does, a rubber ring can be used to sit on, or the baby can be fed while you lie on your side. Gentle pelvic floor exercises help to get the muscles back to normal. Infra-red irradiation or the application of ultrasound may be used to diminish swelling and bruising. At home, even a hairdryer is comforting, or the midwife may suggest an ice pack.'

Induction

Why? 'It is usually because the baby is overdue and you are sure that your dates are correct. If in doubt, ultrasound can be used to estimate the baby's size. Sometimes it is because the baby is large, and sometimes because pre-eclampsia is developing.' The class may need to be reminded of the signs of pre-eclampsia.

How is it done? 'You will be admitted into hospital one afternoon for induction the next day. After a very early breakfast or just a cup of tea, a sedative injection is given some time in the morning, and you will go to the labour ward. The injection gives a peaceful relaxed feeling. On the labour ward bed, slings will be used to arrange your legs in an open position.' If a teacher feels she has the confidence to demonstrate the lithotomy position herself, she should do so, explaining that the legs can feel quite comfortable as they are well supported. She can discuss embarrassment and suggest that the whole thing is routine to the doctors and nurses, and that the class should try to think themselves into this attitude too, and accept with relaxation.

'As there are often a few minutes in this position, and you will be going to have a vaginal examination, practise vaginal tightening and releasing, so that the vagina can be relaxed when the doctor is ready. He will put a small instrument into the vagina and gently up through the cervix, usually telling you what he is doing. Then with pressure he breaks the waters (this is also called rupturing the membranes, or a surgical induction). If the vagina is relaxed and you concentrate on gentle upper-chest breathing, it should feel just like pressure, and not painful. The water, or liquor, will feel warm as it flows out.

'Sometimes a drip will be set up at the same time, or there may be an hour or so's waiting to see if labour begins. You have all seen pictures on television of the drip stand with the bottle upside down and a tube running to a vein in the arm. A small needle is inserted, usually in a vein at the wrist, and the tube attached to it. Apart from the prick when the needle goes in the drip should be painless, and the needle is covered with a piece of plaster or a bandage so you don't have to look at it. The liquid in the bottle is a mixture of sterile water, glucose and a special hormone. This hormone builds up normally in the last weeks of pregnancy and is one of the triggers of labour. By putting extra hormone into the body, contractions usually start quickly, fairly close together, and build up rapidly in length and strength. The drip alone may be used if the membranes rupture spontaneously and contractions do not begin. A less usual way of giving the hormone is in tablet form. It will be destroyed by the stomach acids if swallowed, so you will be asked to place it at the side of your mouth between your cheek and upper gums. Here it is slowly absorbed by glands. Half a tablet is given first, then in half-hour intervals, a whole tablet, sometimes increasing to two to three tablets, still with half-hour spaces. When labour begins the tablets have to be kept in the mouth until the contractions are strong and regular.

'As the "drip" works quicker, it is usually the favoured method. However, labour can be very speedy once started in this way, and some obstetricians and anaesthetists offer a "package deal" of the drip followed by epidural analgesia when the contractions become strong, as strong lengthy contractions coming suddenly can be difficult to tolerate without this help'.

What good or harm can it do? 'A quicker labour is often thought to be better for both mother and baby. It is much better than allowing you to be very overdue or pre-eclampsia to develop—in fact, it helps to ensure a healthier baby. A minor disadvantage, from the mother's point of view, is that you may have to stay in bed for the whole of your labour, and any movements in bed will be somewhat restricted.'

A method of preinduction is being used now in some hospitals. A prostaglandin gel is inserted through the cervix in the evening and will slowly 'ripen' and thin a thick cervix ready for an easier labour the next day. Midwives have a system of estimating the length, thickness and tightness of the cervix, which is named the 'Bishops score'. Points are given from one to ten and a thin cervix, slightly dilated already (as often happens with multipara) would be given a score of ten. Usually, if the score is five or less, the gel is used. The gel is now also being made into a small pessary, so that none of it is wasted in the vagina, or is given orally. The technique can be explained as follows:

'You are already in hospital, waiting for an induction. In the evening a midwife examines you vaginally, to see how thick the cervix is.' (This can be demonstrated with the Birth Atlas.) 'If it is still fairly thick, she will put a small pessary through the cervix, or squeeze out some gel into the uterus. This is a hormone called prostaglandin. She then, if the gel is used, asks you to stay in bed for at least an hour, so that the gel doesn't slip out into the vagina.

During this hour, the baby's heartbeat may be monitored, and will certainly be checked regularly. This is because the baby's heart-rate sometimes changes due to the hormones in your body. As we have said before, whatever is in your bloodstream will go to some extent to the baby. After this hour, you can settle down. You may be offered a sleeping tablet, and should get a good night's sleep.

In the morning, it is possible that labour will have already started, especially with second or subsequent babies. If not, the cervix will be thinner and softer.'

What does it feel like? 'Just like an ordinary vaginal examination. Remember to relax while being examined.'

What good or harm can it do? 'Certainly no harm. It may prevent a full scale induction altogether. If it doesn't the labour is quicker, as the thin cervix gives the induction a good start.'

Some obstetricians prefer the prostaglandins to be given by mouth in tablet form, and some inject them into a vein, as in an ordinary induction.

Obstetric staff will know that induction is not now performed as frequently as in the past year or two, and also that other refinements of the techniques are being introduced. In some hospitals, the contractions and fetal heart rate are measured (as on p. 112) and when good 'peaking' of contractions occurs (even, strong contractions with three or four minutes between them) the drip is turned down. It has been found that often, even with less hormone given, the contractions will continue at this strength, and not get short and colicky, occurring faster, as is usually the case with the oxytocin continuing at the same strength. The drip can then be turned down again, and the oxytocin may be able to be turned off, leaving a glucose drip for nourishment only. The contractions continue in the same pattern, are easier for a patient to handle than the short, sharp colicky ones, and are more effective in dilating the cervix.

We mention this variation, not to be taught in classes unless questions are asked, but to demonstrate how speedily changes are being made in obstetrics. This means that a teacher should try to keep abreast of the changes by visiting hospitals when possible, and certainly by reading current journals.

A very short labour

Why is it happening? 'Nobody really knows why some women have speedy labours. It seems sometimes to follow a mother-daughter pattern, and certainly a woman who has had one fast labour should prepare herself for it to happen the next time. A long first labour does not mean a repeat of this the second time however.'

What will it feel like? 'The contractions will start with short intervals, which rapidly get shorter still and the contractions longer. Great concentration is needed to keep up the relaxing and breathing techniques, and pain relief should be accepted early, as the labour seems to be too fast to catch the contractions and deal with them properly.

'Usually, in a fast labour, the baby is in a beautiful position for birth, and suffers no harm from his speedy entry into the world. Unless you have great control at delivery you will usually have to have stitches due to the speed of the birth itself.

A very long labour

'Again, usually the cause is not definite, but it can happen because the baby is not in a perfect position, and the contractions have to turn him into the correct position for birth. The contractions themselves may be weak, short and far apart. A full bladder or a full rectum can both lengthen labour because the baby's head hasn't enough space to curve round the birth canal.'

How does it feel? 'It feels boring, tedious and very tiring. Concentration on breathing and relaxation techniques become difficult because of tiredness, and again some analgesia should be accepted gladly, this time for a rest. As most hospitals don't allow food when labour is well established, hunger adds to the tiredness. Sometimes a glucose drip is put up to give energy. In the second stage you may have become too tired to push effectively and forceps may be used for the delivery.'

Precipitate labour

'Again, nobody knows why this happens. It has been suggested that a woman may have such a high pain threshold that she just doesn't notice labour until second stage. Needless to say, this is very, very rare. Women to whom this has happened say that, after a few abdominal cramps, they feel like having their bowels opened, then realise they are in labour as the feeling comes in waves.'

How to help oneself. 'Send somebody—anybody—for an ambulance or the doctor if he's near. Keep somebody at home. Lie down— if on the bed, on old sheeting or newspaper if some is handy. Whenever a contraction comes, pant like a dog on a hot day—hard. Probably help will arrive. If it doesn't, keep panting as the head is born, being assured that a quick delivery like this is going to be normal. With the next contraction give a little push, and the whole baby will be born. Ask whoever is with you to hold the baby upside down and wipe his mouth out thoroughly with a clean handkerchief. If he is not yelling, tickle his back. When he is crying well, hold him in your arms (the cord will stretch to allow this) and have your helper wrap you and the baby up warmly. Wait for help. If the afterbirth or placenta comes out, just leave it. These quick labours only happen once in a million or so births and even then usually with a mother who has had several children and "knows the ropes" anyway.'

What harm can come to mother or child? 'The mother may have to have stitches. The baby is not harmed at all, so long as his mouth can be cleaned properly so that he can cry, and then he is kept warm.'

At the Third International Congress of Psychosomatic Medicine in Obstetrics and Gynaecology in London in 1971 a paper was given by Dr J. S. Sambhi about Malaysian women who have this type of labour. He called them 'Short and Sweet Labours'.

Cessation or slowing of contractions

I have just referred to the 1971 Congress. In the same Congress a paper was given on the effect of handling mice once labour had been established, and of moving them from place to place in labour. On all occasions labour was interrupted, the contractions ceasing for some time. Professor Niles Newton, of the Department of Psychiatry, Northwestern University Medical School, who gave the paper, equated this with the interruption of contractions which often happens when a woman moves from home to hospital.

'Sometimes you get ready to go to hospital with contractions strong and regular, yet while travelling there they stop. This may be a false alarm, but more often they stop until the strangeness of the hospital wears off, and you begin to feel at home, they then begin again and are soon as regular as they were before. If this happens to you, don't worry. Be thankful that you can have your bath in peace. Accept your pattern.

'Sometimes the contractions become weaker and the intervals between them longer, when you have been in good labour for a considerable time. The cause *may* be a full bladder, or the position of the baby, but is more likely to be tiredness. A strong sedative may be given to allow restful sleep, and labour will then carry on when you are refreshed, or the uterus may be stimulated by putting up a drip. The only frustration of the sedative is having to accept everything slowing down. The drip, however, may produce sudden rapid contractions. In any case, try to accept that this is the way your labour is going, remembering that everyone is different.'

Fetal reactions to labour

Fetal heart monitoring. 'We have already mentioned the abdominal disc which can be attached to a machine and records the baby's heartbeat (p. 91). Actually, the machine, when attached for most of the end of labour, can do more than we stated, as its use is now not to count the baby's heartbeats only, but also to draw on the same piece of paper a pattern of contractions. A light, usually a pulsating green light, is also continuously recording the baby's heart rate. If you wish it, the midwife will turn a switch and let you hear the baby's heart sounds, which are quite loud, but very reassuring. She does not keep the sound on, as the light and the tracing tell her all she needs to know. Please remind your husband beforehand that he will be in the labour ward to be your companion and support, and not to watch the machine (we always make this point in parents' classes, as husbands tend to be fascinated by machinery). There are some snags in monitoring the baby's heart like this. It is possible that you could hear the midwives say. "The heart sound is gone". *Don't panic!* This usually means that either you or the baby has changed position, and it is difficult, certainly, for you to keep lying in one position, and not advisable. The movement, however, sometimes disturbs the disc from the position over baby's heart. There is no reason for the baby to stay completely still either, and often he turns a little. However, after adjusting the position of the disc once or twice, the midwife may decide that a more reliable method of monitoring the heart is needed.

'She does a vaginal examination, and, even with the cervix only slightly open, can fix what is called a 'fetal electrode' to the baby's head. Of course, the membranes have to be broken, or she couldn't feel the head. The electrode looks a bit like a tube with a thicker end and she presses this to the baby's scalp. A tiny hook catches the baby's skin, which will result later in a very tiny scab, like a small spot on the head. Now, you and the baby can both move, and the tracings will continue. The tube goes to the machine and is usually fixed to your leg with a bit of sticking plaster.

'Some hospitals, instead of having the elastic band with the disc, round your abdomen, put a small tube into the uterus to record your contractions. The two tubes are then attached together to the machine and you are even more mobile. In fact, recently, a small battery-operated transmitter has been designed so that there is no need, when these are available, to be physically attached to the machine at all. The two tubes are fixed together, and fitted to the transmitter, which can be carried in a shoulder bag or in a pocket. This means that women can walk around in labour and be completely free, as the transmitter can relay all information back to the machine from a distance of up to 200 metres. Many women like to walk around in labour, and indeed, obstetricians believe that this mobility often shortens the labour, and also makes the mother feel much happier. These mobile transmitters are only used in a very few places at present, but their use is regarded with interest by the medical profession, and more are becoming available. (Flynn et al., 1978) Mobile monitoring is called radio-telemetry.

Hospitals which encourage mobility in labour but have not yet got radio-telemetry, are now using monitoring machines as soon as each woman is admitted in labour. The bands recording the contractions and the fetal heart are placed round her abdomen, and kept on for a period of fifteen to twenty minutes. The graph can be compared with further short periods of recording as labour continues, and between these recordings the bands are removed and complete freedom of movement is maintained.

Sonic Aid monitoring. The Sonic Aid is like a small stethoscope, which can record the baby's heartbeat by touching the abdomen. Unlike a stethoscope, however, the other end does not have to be in anyone's ears. The noise of the baby's heart is amplified, and you and your partner will be able to hear it also. Sonic Aids are useful when you want to keep changing positions, as the midwife can usually touch the abdomen with it, whatever position you choose.

It is a good way of remaining mobile, and yet knowing that the baby is being monitored.

Fetal blood sampling. Very occasionally a small amount of blood may be removed from the baby's scalp. This assesses the acid/base balance and glucose level of its blood and the doctor can estimate how fit or tired the baby is.

Posterior positions

A suitable floppy doll should be used to show, against the teacher's own body, the different anterior and posterior positions. The turning of the head to achieve the occipito-frontal position for birth then makes it obvious that a baby lying anteriorly will have to turn little, while a baby lying posteriorly has to make a turn of almost half a circle, and flex his head much more in doing so.

As the baby is turned, something like this can be said:

'You can see it's going to take the baby a bit longer to make the bigger movements. This isn't up to the baby at all—the contractions push him round, and he can help no more than a passenger on a train can make it go faster. So labour may be longer, but with effective contractions this isn't always so. There may be a lot of backache with each contraction. Someone should know how to do back massage effectively to ease this ache, or epidural analgesia may be advised. Occasionally the baby doesn't turn completely. In this case you wouldn't feel much like pushing in second stage, and the pushing would be ineffective as the head would be in the wrong position to come through the vagina. The doctor will turn the head to the right position and with his help you can push it out.

'Sometimes, if you have a nice roomy pelvis, or one which is wider towards the back, the head can turn towards the back and be born' (demonstrate). 'Instead of a glimpse of the back of his head at birth, his face will be in front. This is called a face-to-pubes delivery' (point to the position of the pubic bone).

Breech positions

The doll is again used to show the different positions arms and legs can achieve in a breech birth.

'Many hospitals insist that if you have a breech delivery you spend most of your labour in bed. This is to try to prevent the waters from breaking early. Labour proceeds normally, but the aching and pressure with contractions may be less, as the buttocks are softer than the head. Once the waters break (membranes rupture) you very soon feel like pushing, because the soft body or a leg of the baby can easily begin to come through a cervix which has only partially opened. You will be told not to push until the cervix becomes fully dilated, and it is often difficult to stop. For this reason many doctors recommend epidural analgesia for all breech births.

'When pushing begins the baby's legs and buttocks are soon born (a bonus—the sex is identified!). You keep on pushing until the shoulders are born, then the doctor takes over and delivers the head slowly and carefully by forceps. He doesn't want the head to be born too quickly. You remember how a baby's head changes shape as it is born, and a head-first baby does this slowly, so he gives the head a little time to change shape, so that the baby doesn't have a severe headache after he is born.

'In most cases, when the birth is not completely straightforward the baby is nursed in a special-care nursery for up to 48 hours. This depends on the tiredness of the baby and also on the routine of the hospital. Some hospitals will keep every baby in this nursery after a forceps delivery even if obviously not tired.

'The snags are the difficulty in stopping pushing until full dilatation of the cervix, the use of forceps which usually means more stitches, and the frustration of seeing the other mothers with their babies beside them shortly after birth. The delivery itself should not be painful: if you have been given epidural analgesia there will be no pain; if not, you will either have local anaesthesia all round the vagina or a brief complete anaesthesia for the forceps delivery.

'If you have already given birth to a child you could, probably, with your stretchable vagina, push the head out without the use of forceps.'

'With a first baby, the doctor may decide to do a Caesarean section, as these are now very safe, and much more common today.' (See Caesarean section.)

A forceps delivery

'We have already discussed several reasons for a forceps delivery— a breech birth, a long labour, a tired baby and a posterior position where the baby hasn't quite turned properly. Another reason is that the second stage, even with the baby in a perfect position, is taking too long. Most obstetricians don't like you to have the effort of pushing for longer than an hour, and prefer to lift it out.'

How is it done? (Differences between hospitals must be known.) 'Sometimes a light general anaesthetic is given by an injection in the arm, and you wake to find the forceps delivery completed and the baby giving his first cry. Sometimes the obstetrician gives the nerve-blocking local anaesthetic. Although several injections are needed for this, usually only the first one is felt. He waits a little until the perineum and vagina are numb,then slips the forceps round the baby's head and locks them so that they fit round the head smoothly. They are like two hands' (someone holds the doll upside down and the teacher slides her hands up and round its head) 'and are placed round the head like this. It's easy to see now how the head can be turned to a good position. Often with the next contraction you feel a terrific urge to push and are told to go ahead. As you push, the doctor guides the baby's head out.'

What will if feel like?   'With a general anaesthetic—nothing. And the anaesthetic is so light that one doesn't feel sick afterwards. With a local anaesthetic—a dull feeling of pulling.' This can be discussed, especially if someone in class has already had the experience and can describe it.

What good or harm will it do to me or my baby?   'To get a tired baby out before he ges more tired can do nothing but good; he will revive quicker and be healthier. He may have small red pressure marks on his head, but these will quickly disappear. He may be placed in the special-care nursery at first.

'From the mother's point of view, as a forceps delivery is quicker than a normal second stage and as the forceps stretch the vagina more, there is always an episiotomy, almost certainly more stitches than with a normal delivery, and sometimes more bruising. This always seems more painful on the second and third days after delivery, and the stitches pull whenever one moves quickly. The nurses will advise lots of baths, sometimes with salt in the water, which, surprisingly, are enormously soothing'.

Ventouse vacuum extraction

This technique of delivery appears to be used very little at the present time, but it should be briefly mentioned, in case some members of the class have heard of it, or meet somebody in hospital who has been delivered in this manner.

Why is it used?   'It is used for all the reasons that forceps are used, except a breech delivery—a long labour, a tired baby or mother, a baby who hasn't turned through the birth canal properly, or a long second stage. It can be used earlier than forceps though, with the head higher, and sometimes when the cervix isn't quite open.'

How is it used?   'You have all seen the rubber suction cups which stick on the kitchen wall to hold teatowels. Imagine a suction cup made of metal, and attached by a rubber tube to a machine which can keep up the vacuum inside it. The cup is quite small. The doctor first numbs the vagina and perineum with a local anaesthetic, then puts the cup into the vagina and presses it against the baby's head. The vacuum is built up gently, and the cup fits tightly on the baby's head. Now, whenever a contraction comes, the doctor can help the baby to be born quicker by turning the cup if the head position is not perfect, and pulling a little at the correct angle. With each contraction, mother and doctor cooperate, and the baby is born fairly quickly, but not so speedily as with forceps'.

What does it feel like? 'As a local anaesthetic is used, there is no pain as the cup is fitted. After this, it doesn't touch the mother, only the baby's head, but with each contraction there is a sensation of being helped to push more effectively, and a slight feeling of pulling. That is all. As soon as the widest part of the head is born, the vacuum is released, the cup drops off, and the baby is born normally.

'The main snag is that, although the cup doesn't damage the head at all, the suction pulls the baby's scalp into the shape of the cup, so that when the baby is born he has a round bump like a chignon or bun on his head. This lasts for a week or two in some cases, but does no harm. Many babies have round bumps on their heads with normal labours, anyway, simply by being pressed against the cervix. These usually disappear in a few days, as the "vacuum babies" buns might do also. Just as with any other interference, of course, the baby may have to stay longer in the special nursery.'

Caesarean section

Why is it done? 'The main reasons are because the baby is too big or the pelvis too small for the head to fit in properly, bleeding before labour begins, difficult positions of the baby, a long labour, or a tired baby when it's too early to do a forceps delivery or a vacuum extraction. You can see that these are all good reasons, and if a Caesarean section isn't done a healthy baby won't be born. No woman particularly wants a "Caesar", but will put up with it for the reward of a healthy baby.'

How is it done? 'A surprisingly small cut is made through the abdomen, usually what is called a "bikini cut", in the fold of skin just above the pubic hair. This means that the scar will be almost invisible when healed. The uterus is opened and the baby delivered, then everything is stitched up again. It takes a surprisingly short time and is a very safe operation.'

How will it feel? 'There are two main methods of making Caesarean sections painless today. The first is like any routine operation. An injection is given to make the woman feel sleepy and her mouth becomes dry. Then she is taken to theatre and an injection into a vein in her arm sends her to sleep in a few seconds. She wakes, feeling very drowsy, to be told she has a son or a daughter, and probably goes to sleep again immediately. The baby is taken to the special care nursery to be observed, he may be tired, as the rapid delivery may have been preceeded by a labour, but babies are resilient, and he usually recovers quickly.

'The second method is never used unless the mother wishes it, and is not available in all hospitals. This is delivery with epidural analgesia (i.e. local anaesthesia in the epidural space, as previously described). Some women, knowing they will be awake, are afraid in case they have sudden pain; this does not happen.

'If she chooses epidural analgesia, she usually has an injection first to make her feel comfortably relaxed. Then the epidural drip is set up, as described, and, when working well, the operation begins. A screen is put up so that the woman cannot see her actual abdomen, but can see the doctors' faces. A nurse usually sits by the patient, and holds her hand, although recently in many hospitals fathers have taken over this role. In a very short time, the baby is heard to cry, and is put into his mother's arms by a midwife. One woman observed, 'I was waiting, feeling rather scared, for the first cut, when I felt a slight pulling, heard a squelching sound, and the baby was in my arms. I couldn't believe it!''

'She can cuddle her baby while the stitching of the small cut is being done, then the baby has a rest. As the epidural wears off she is given an injection for the returning sensation and pain, as with a general anaesthetic procedure, but it appears that less pain relief is required than after a Caesarean section with an ordinary anaesthetic.

'In a normal labour, pain has vanished when the baby is born, except for stitch discomfort. After a Caesarean section a woman sleeps with strong sedatives for the first 12 hours or so, then these are replaced by pain-relieving tablets, which do not take away all discomfort. At the same time the physiotherapist will encourage her to breathe deeply and to cough, and this will be uncomfortable. On the second and third days the abdomen feels full of wind, and this is not very pleasant as it seems to be pressing on the scar. Also, within 24 hours, she gets out of bed, which takes some effort and pain. However, very soon she can be pushed in a wheelchair to see her baby in the nursery, which makes the effort worth while. Usually in a short time she can have her baby with her and breastfeed him if she wants to. By the fourth day she is feeling much better, and will be encouraged by the physiotherapists to walk with a straight back. She may then find it easier to walk and sit than the women who have had lots of stitches after a normal labour. However, a Caesarean is an operation, not a normal body function, so she will have to stay in hospital for up to 12 days, and will need gradual convalescence at home, and much more help in the house than after a normal delivery.'

TWINS

A teacher should be ready to answer questions, and may be asked about the differences in labour in the births of twins. A facile answer would be 'Two for the price of one', but if a member of the class is suspected of carrying twins, or knows she is, details of extra rest in pregnancy, perhaps in hospital, and the possibility of premature births, should be given. A brief description could follow, of the one first stage to open the cervix, and second stage and delivery of the first infant, then the abdominal, and perhaps vaginal examination to define the presenting part of the second twin. One should describe how the uterus rests before contractions begin again—usually for anything up to half an hour—then another second stage and delivery. The *Birth Atlas* gives a good pictorial explanation of how identical twins are proved, showing clearly the sharing of the chorion of the membranes, while each infant has his own amniotic sac.

RETAINED PLACENTA

Occasionally retained placenta will be mentioned, usually because 'it happened to a friend'. One can remind the class of the injection given, at the time of birth, into the mother's thigh, and reassure them that this injection has cut down the numbers of retained placentas to a very small number indeed. However, the simplicity of removal under a light general anaesthetic can be stressed, although perhaps it should be mentioned that if much blood is lost it will be replaced by a blood transfusion. One can emphasise that a transfusion does not mean serious illness, but merely a quick way of making a woman feel fit again.

DIFFERENCES IN HOSPITAL BOOKINGS

A teacher should be aware of the types of care available in her area, for pregnancy, labour and the puerperium, as women often wish to discuss and compare differences in class. Each area is somewhat different, and if a class group is attending several hospitals, there will be many variants. Here are a few.

Pregnancy

From the date of making the hospital booking, the staff there may wish to give all care. Some hospitals share care with the family doctor, if he is willing to do this, so that, without complications, a woman would only have to attend hospital three or four times during the pregnancy. Occasionally after booking the hospital, the family doctor may take all responsibility for care. She is routinely seen also by her health visitor in all these cases, and will be seen at home by the domiciliary midwife if she wants an early discharge after the birth. In some areas now, domiciliary midwives visit all pregnant women.

Labour

Usually, the mother is looked after by the hospital midwives and doctors. However, with shared antenatal care, the GP may attend her in labour with the midwives. He will then be at the delivery when possible.

If a woman has had one baby with no complications, she may wish to have the baby at home, in which case, she would be attended by the domiciliary midwives and her own doctor, who must have given consent to take over responsibility, although the midwives conduct the majority of the labour. Home deliveries are becoming rarer since the advent of the 'Domino' scheme, but at least one hospital is conducting a survey to study and compare home and hospital confinements in terms of safety, the effect on family relationships, and cost effectiveness.

Puerperium

Overall responsibility may be taken by the hospital, or, with shared care, by the family doctor. With the 'Domino' scheme, mother and baby will be quickly home, cared for by the domiciliary midwives and their doctor. The mother may have chosen to go home after 48 hours, when the care is as above.

If not, the hospital policy may be to keep the mother and baby in for ten days, but earlier discharge is more usual—from six to nine days. Until recently, the health visitor then was reponsible for advice, but now with more midwives, the midwife will care for the family for at least the first ten days, leaving her telephone number for 24-hour calls. After this, the health visitor arrives, but the midwives inform the mother that if she needs advice when the health visitor is not obtainable, they can be called in until the baby is 28 days old (Central Midwives Board rules).

The Domino Scheme

This perhaps has the best of both worlds. A teacher should find out if local hospitals have developed Domiciliary Midwife Units in hospital, where a multigravida can have her hospital period cut to a very short time indeed. These units may be called short-stay units, or DOMINO, i.e. DOMiciliary, IN, Out.

A fairly typical routine is that, on having pregnancy confirmed, her general practitioner assesses the multigravida's health and obstetric history, decides that she is fit and checks that she had normal pregnancies previously. He then asks her to see her district midwife, who 'books' her as she would a patient to be delivered at home, and considers the suitability of the home and the help available after the birth. All the patient's notes then are sent to the hospital, again checked, and a bed is reserved in the unit. Throughout pregnancy her antenatal examinations are carried out by her general practitioner and her midwife. When she begins labour she calls the midwife, who cares for her at home until labour is well advanced, then takes her to hospital by ambulance. There she delivers her (although the general practitioner may also be present and may do the delivery) and stays to bath the baby and make the mother comfortable. When she leaves, the hospital provides 'hotel service' of meals and care. A few hours later the midwife returns, baths the mother and takes the mother and baby home again by ambulance, where she continues to nurse them both exactly as if it had been a home delivery.

One can see at once that this is almost a home delivery, and therefore acceptable to the mother, but if any obstetric or paediatric emergency should arise, all the hospital facilities are immediately available.

It appears that Domino schemes are not increasing in the country as a whole. Instead, all patients are encouraged to choose the length of stay which they feel they will prefer. If this is to be shorter than eight days, the domiciliary midwife will call to see them during pregnancy, and then continue to care for them when they are discharged with their babies. A primigravida can choose a short stay if she wishes—anything over 48 hours—and be home with her midwife, just as the multigravida has been able to do in the past. In fact, many hospitals are making a short stay routine for all patients, unless complications have arisen, which means that all of them meet the midwife at home during pregnancy. This saves expensive hospital care, and allows all the pregnant women to talk to a midwife in their own homes, which is much better than in a busy antenatal clinic.

It does pre-suppose adequate home care by relatives, which is not always possible, and also a well-staffed domiciliary unit attached to each hospital.

There is also the problem of continuity of care. An experiment to achieve this is in progress at St George's Hospital, London, under the guidance of Caroline Flint (see Films—'A Question of Confidence') Small teams of three to four midwives are being formed, who are getting to know each mother. Once a mother has been allocated to a team, they will take care of her antenatally, with advice from a consultant as necessary. One of them will visit her at home, and one of the team will be with her in labour and stay until the baby is born, as a community midwife would with a home birth. The team will then continue to visit her at home.

This seems as near 'personal' maternity care as the Health Service can expect to provide, as the other members of the team will dovetail off-duty and holiday periods, and each mother will really know 'her' midwife.

The Maternity Services Advisory Committee (*Maternity Care in Action*, 1982) recommends more personalised maternity care in its report—'the need for good clinical care, sensitive to the emotional needs of the mother, the father, and their other children. All women need a service where their own particular questions and problems are treated sympathetically and in private. Health authorities should look at their present activity, and make the best use of the skills and resources available in hospitals, community services, and general practice, and so provide a more personal and satisfying service.'

We mention these differences to show how a teacher should 'keep pace' with changing methods; probably many other new methods will be initiated in the future and need to be known. Perhaps, as in the U.S.A, home deliveries will almost disappear, or, if surveys are successful, be revived to a much greater extent.

One recent innovation, however, is that whole families are welcomed into the hospital at visiting times in many places. Thus, the family unit can welcome the new baby from birth.

REFERENCES

Bradley, R. A. (1965) *Husband-coached Childbirth*, Ch. 8. New York and London: Harper and Row.
Flynn, A. M. Kelly, J., Hollins, G. & Lynch, P. F. (1978) Ambulation in labour *British Medical Journal*, 2, 591–593.
Kitzinger, S. (ed.) (1980) *Episiotomy—Physical and Emotional Aspects*. London: National Childbirth Trust.

Kitzinger, S., Walters, R. (1981) *Some Women's Experiences of Episiotomy.* London: National Childbirth Trust.
Maternity Care in Action (1982) Part 1. Antenatal care. London: Maternity Services Advisory Committee.

FURTHER READING

Brynon, C. (1974) Midline episiotomy as a routine procedure. *The Journal of Obstetrics and Gynaecology of the British Commonwealth*, **81**, 126–30.
Donovan, B. (1978) *The Caesarean Birth Experience.* Obtainable I.C.E.A.
Hickman, M. (1978) *An Introduction to Midwifery.* London: Blackwood Scientific Publications
Hoare, S. & Weig, M. *Episiotomy.* A Birth Centre London Leaflet.
National Childbirth Trust Leaflets (1977) No. 12 *Episiotomy: What Happens when Labour is Induced*; No. 13 *How to Cope with a Caesarean Section.*
Reading, A. E., Sledmere, C. M., Cox, D. N. & Campbell, S. (1982) How women view post-episiotomy pain. *British Medical Journal*, **284**, 243–245.
Sweet, B. & Cape, I. (1976) In *Nursing Modules. Obstetric Care.* London: H. M. & M.

8

Some new ideas

Something of the 'active birth' movement both here and abroad has already been described, and alternative positions for the first stage of labour mentioned. Here are some further details of how the second stage may be managed in units where the technique is practised, and also some new ideas on breathing in labour.

THE 'ACTIVE' SECOND STAGE

In all primitive communities, women give birth in a semi-upright position. All drawings, paintings and sculptures of birth, from ancient history up to the eighteenth century, show this upright posture.

In Egypt around 2500 BC, women sat on birth stools. Hippocrates wrote of the use of a birth stool or chair in labour. The first chapter of Exodus refers to birth stools (and to midwives) in verses 15 and 16.

The Israel Department of Antiquities Museum has a statuette in Cypriot clay of a group of three women, dated 8 BC, with the labouring woman supported on each side by attendants, so that she is in a semi-squatting position.

Throughout Europe, birth stools were commonly used in the Middle Ages.

Why did we change to a dorsal (or, as is inelegantly expressed, a 'stranded beetle' posture?)

One theory is that it began because Louis XIV of France wanted to see his mistress, Madame de Montespan, actually giving birth to his child, and as he was watching from behind a curtain, she had to be flat.

More probably, it was because, at about this time, the Chamberlain brothers in France invented obstetric forceps, which could only be used with a woman lying down. At this time, obstetricians began to take over from midwives and, for their convenience, the birthing stool became the labour bed.

In the nineteenth century, when Queen Victoria used chloroform, it became fashionable, and with the spread of anaesthesia and analgesia, sitting or squatting was obviously not possible, and lying down became the norm in Europe, and also in America, even though the shape and direction of the birth canal meant pushing against gravity.

Midwives delivering at home were still encouraging mobility, especially in Holland, where home birth is still routine in normal pregnancy.

Recently, continuous monitoring of contractions and the fetal heart has meant that women have not only been forced to lie down, but also to keep still, and to stay in bed for most of their labours.

At the Active Birth Conference in Wembley (October, 1982) Dr Marsden Wagner, of the World Health Organization, said 'The mechanisation of birth makes a woman into a machine to which other machines can be attached.'

America went to extremes—midwifery was no longer a profession, and obstetricians, trained to surgical operations, made birth into a surgical procedure.

In the second stage, the woman's legs were held high in stirrups, while her wrists were fastened to the bed with straps to avoid touching the 'sterile area'.

In the U.K., obstetricians made policy rules, but normal birth was still the province of the midwife, and birth was never as strictly controlled as this. Still, until recently, midwives were being trained to be machine-oriented, for the 'safety of the baby'.

The growth of the feminist movement in America made women look at their behaviour, and the 'free' sixties made them react against this rigid hospital procedure. In effect, some women said, 'Here we are, as women, doing something which no man can do, and yet surrendering all the power and triumph of this act into a man's hands.'

In Tennessee and California, where women were living with their men in communes, some of them decided to do without doctors and deliver each other. Although illegal, there had always been a few 'granny' midwives in America, practising in poor communities, and the women learned from them, from each other, and from textbooks. As they had no drugs, they had to find methods of easing pain, and began again to move about, change positions, use massage, and in the second stage to squat, lean forwards on a support, or push the baby out on hands and knees.

Some of the positions were similar to the ones used in Holland. At the Active Birth Conference, Beatrice Smulders, a midwife from the Netherlands, told of the simple preparations made at home for a birth. She showed a film of a home delivery, with a midwife and a maternity aid nurse working together. In this film, a strong bucket was placed in front of the mother's armchair, lined with a thick towel. She balanced, with the aid of her husband and nurse, in a semi-squatting position on the edge of the chair and the bucket, while the midwife delivered the baby. The delivery looked homely and comfortable, with, as Ms Smulders said, the midwife 'inspiring the mother to give birth with her own strength and harmony'.

Here, in the U.K., we have never lost our midwives. Some of them reacted strongly against the mechanisation of normal birth, and founded the Association of Radical Midwives in 1976 (see p. 261).

At the same time, Dr Caldeyro-Barcia, in Brazil, was conducting trials which proved that an upright position in the second stage leads to fewer but more effective and stronger contractions (see refs.).

In France, Dr Michel Odent was publicising his ideas of 'instinctive birth', where he found that, if given loving companionship and freedom from fear, a woman would harmonise with her body. Again, the labouring woman adopted an upright position in the second stage of labour.

Obstetricians became interested in the findings of Caldeyro-Barcia and Odent, and began to adopt their work in their own hospitals. One of the first was Dr Faith Haddad, at the West London Hospital. At first, she helped women to give birth kneeling, semi-squatting with support, or on mattresses on the floor (see Fig. 14). She encouraged any second stage position which was comfortable and effective, except lying flat. Her enthusiasm and good results culminated in the West London Hospital obtaining enough money from charities to buy 'borning beds' from America, where the concept of upright second stage had spread to hospitals.

These beds can be manipulated by the woman, her partner, or the midwife, to give comfortable support in almost any position— for instance, sitting upright, with half the bed lowered to allow an 'armchair' position, kneeling with armrests, or squatting with support. With these versatile beds, the midwife remains close to the mother, and can deliver the baby without contorting herself into uncomfortable positions.

However, these beds are expensive, and other hospitals have found different ways of allowing freedom of movement with support. Some have bought 'Kings Fund' beds, which can be lowered and tilted. Other beds are now being made such as the St. Mary's labour ward bed. Some have put mattresses on the floor, and

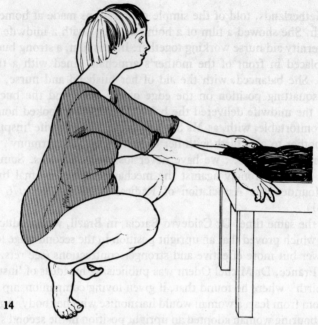

Fig. 14

others have obtained 'Birthing Stools'. (Fig. 15). One London hospital has followed the Dutch method, provided easy chairs, and asked mothers to bring their own buckets with them if they found the position on the bucket comfortable, when practising antenatally.

So the position for the second stage is no longer static. The baby can still be monitored—even with a contraction band while sitting in a chair—but in any position the mother chooses by the use of a Sonic Aid.

To be able to be active in the second stage, it is best if a woman has remained supple, has strengthened her muscles and joints, especially her hips, knees and ankles, and has practised the positions in pregnancy.

However, this is not absolutely essential.

Upright birth has proved so effective and efficient that midwives are now encouraging women to change to semi-squatting or kneeling if pushing is ineffective lying down or sitting. They are providing lots of pillows and a firm wedge to allow all women to sit up in second stage (Fig. 16).

The midwives are enthusiastic. (There were over 1000 midwives at the Active Birth Conference). This makes Active Birth different from other techniques, which often did not have the midwives' full support and encouragement. With psychoprophylaxis, the mother

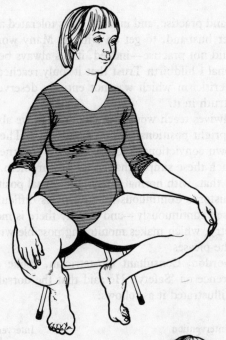

Fig. 15

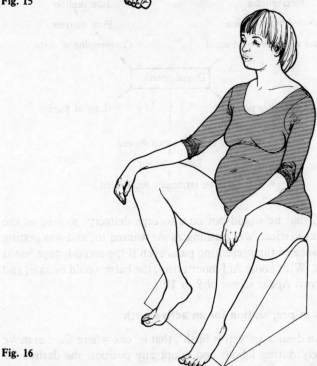

Fig. 16

had to train and practise, and in labour was tolerated and sometimes left, with her husband, to get on with it. Many women were not trained, or did not practise—indeed, it has always been a criticism of the National Childbirth Trust that it 'only reached middle-class women'—a criticism which was not entirely deserved, but had a glimmer of truth in it.

Now, midwives teach women in labour to move about, and help them into upright positions in the second stage. They are doing it from their own convictions, because they have learned by observation how much these simple changes of posture help.

It appears that, with normal births, the dorsal position may soon be part of history. Continuous monitoring is difficult—sonic aids cannot be used continuously—and already there is more interest in radio-telemetry, which makes monitoring possible with the woman moving as she pleases.

Yehudi Gordon, Consultant Obstetrician, spoke at the Active Birth Conference on 'Safety'. He said that the dorsal position was unsafe, and illustrated it as follows:

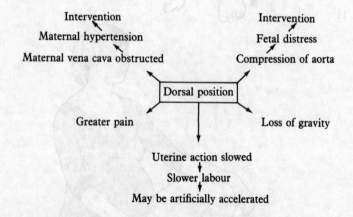

He said that he would not do a forceps delivery, so long as the woman was vertical, was pushing as *she* wanted to, and was getting some advance of the presenting part, even if the second stage lasted two hours. With Sonic Aid monitoring, the baby would be safe, and would record Apgar scores of 9 or 10.

Exercises in preparation for an active birth

If a woman desires an 'active birth', that is, one where she can move about freely during labour and adopt any position she desires for delivery, she will need some preparation beforehand. It will not be possible until the time comes, to know what movements or positions she is going to find most comfortable so she needs to practise all the common ones; these will include standing and sitting, resting forward onto the arms, kneeling and knee chest positions and all the variations of partial and total squatting. We must aim for a mobile spine, hips and feet and strong hip and thigh muscles, since she is often going to hold a position during a contraction.

Exercises should be started early in pregnancy, slowly, and within a comfortable range of movement; no stretching from an outside force should be used since this results in a stretch reflex in which the muscle tends to spring back to its normal length. The present enthusiasm for active birth has led to the recent publication of a number of childbirth exercise books mostly based on Yoga principles, these may be helpful for those who are already doing Yoga classes but should be viewed with suspicion by teachers who have to deal with ordinary, not too fit women during pregnancy.

In addition to the abdominal and pelvic floor exercises and postural and relaxation training already described in this book here is a short list of safe exercises which could be added for those wishing to have an active birth or going to a unit where it may be an option.

1. Pelvic rocking (see p. 97) in all positions but particularly when standing with knees slightly bent, and when kneeling on all fours. The movement can also be done moving the pelvis from side to side and eventually round in a circle like a 'belly dancer'. It is interesting that this essentially sexual movement of native dancing should be so helpful in childbirth.

2. With both feet pointing straightforward take a long stride forward onto the right foot with a bent knee, leave the left heel on the ground and feel the stretch of the calf and the tendon behind the heel. (see Fig. 17)

3. Sit on the ground with the knees open and bent and the soles of the feet together. Place your hands on the *outside* of the knees, then press the knees apart against the pressure of the hands. When the knees won't go any further apart take your hands away and let your legs relax trying to let them fall even further apart. Stay in this position for as long as is possible. (see Fig. 18)

4. Stand with your knees bent to about a right angle, your back against a wall. Maintain the position for a gradually increasing length of time as the weeks go by.

5. Kneel with knees apart facing the seat of an armchair, rest on the forearms for a time, after about a minute collapse down onto

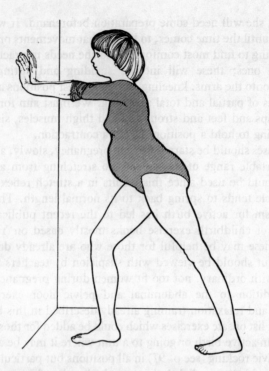

Fig. 17

the floor allowing the head and arms to relax and rest on the chair seat (see Fig. 5, p. 116).

6. Practise a full squat with the heels raised. Gradually increase the length of time you can stay in this position. Not many people are comfortable for long in this posture, though it can be helpful in facilitating the second stage it is not an easy position for delivery for the attendants. Obstetricians who have observed the *full* squat in second stage do not entirely recommend it. At the beginning of this stage it may facilitate the movement of the descending head through the vaginal vault, but as the stage continues, the head has to curve upwards to the vaginal outlet if a full squatting position continues. Mechanically, at this point, a semi-squat with a curved spine, or kneeling forwards with knees well open, uses the directional push through the birth canal much more effectively. Both these positions, with adequate support, can be practised in class. A relaxed modified squat can be very comfortable for the labouring woman though hard work for her helpers. Try a semi-squat with your partner behind you and your arms up and back round his neck, another position would be a semi-squat with a partner kneeling on either side, the mother's arms, right to the arm-pits, being supported by the attendants' shoulders.

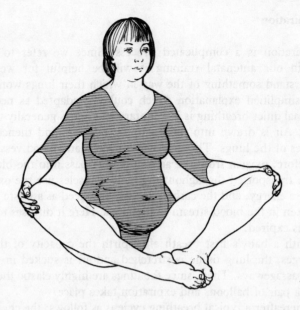

Fig. 18

RESPIRATION IN LABOUR

During the last two years, both here and in the rest of the world, there has been a great deal of discussion about the best kinds of respiration in labour and their possible effects on both mother and baby. Teachers have been alerted by paediatricians, physiologists and psychologists to the dangers of hyperventilation associated with overbreathing and indeed the likelihood of tiring the mother through the imposition on her of any pattern of non-instinctive breathing. It has been pointed out that upper chest breathing is often a sign of tension and anxiety. We are being encouraged to give up teaching levels and rates of breathing which are not physiologically sound in favour of encouraging mothers to use a 'let go and flow' approach (Noble, 1981). On the other hand since we are all human our instincts are sometimes not sufficiently developed to overcome a tendency to become tense and hold our breath in the face of a threat such as a painful uterine contraction, so we still need training to help us to cope with stress.

At the John Radcliffe Hospital, where Sheila Harrison is currently taking part in a study of the effects of hyperventilation, the mothers are first taught a little about the effects of stress on the body (see p. 126) and how to cope with them, then about the mechanics of normal breathing.

Respiration

Respiration is a complicated process. Since we refer to breathing in our antenatal training it will be helpful for women to understand something of the way in which their lungs work. Here is a simplified explanation which could be adapted as necessary. Normal quiet breathing is involuntary and one is generally unaware of it. Air is drawn into the breathing passages and thence to the tissues of the lungs. These tissues contain many blood vessels and, therefore, oxygen from the air can readily pass into the blood and so be transported throughout the body. Muscles use the oxygen to release energy, and the carbon dioxide produced as a waste product is taken in the blood stream to the lungs. Here it diffuses to the air and is expired.

With a baby's first breath after birth the capacity of the chest enlarges, the lung tissue is stretched and air is sucked in through the passageways. Then, since the lungs are highly elastic they recoil like a pair of balloons and expiration takes place.

Thereafter a typical breathing cycle is as follows: the chest cavity enlarges in all directions during inspiration due to movements of the ribs and diaphragm. The latter is a dome-shaped muscle which is attached to the spine and lower ribs, and divides the chest from the abdominal cavity. During inspiration the diaphragm descends like a piston, pushing the abdominal contents forward a little, thus enlarging the vertical dimension of the chest. On expiration the ribs and diaphragm recoil again. The diaphragm is the most important muscle of respiration. If you sit quietly with your eyes shut and place your hands on different parts of your chest as you breathe you will find your breast bone and upper ribs rising and falling gently, your lower ribs expanding sideways and upwards, and your abdomen expanding and contracting a little.

The rhythm of inspiration and expiration, when the body is at rest, is controlled by a centre in the lower part of the brain. This rhythm is fundamentally automatic but can be changed at will or by certain other factors. For example, increased carbon dioxide in the blood causes an increase in the rate and depth of breathing. During strenuous exercise even a healthy person becomes breathless; the point at which this happens varies widely from person to person depending on their 'training' or physical state. If you continue to breathe unusually quickly or deeply for a time a greater than ordinary amount of carbon dioxide is blown from the blood and the respiratory centre does not receive its normal stimulation. When the forced effort ceases, spontaneous respiration may not begin again for as much as two minutes. This state, known as hyperventilation (Lum, 1975), is sometimes seen in women in labour who are breathing too quickly and strongly through fear or pain, or in an attempt to keep control. It is characterised by very quick forced breaths using the upper chest. The woman may feel dizzy or experience pins and needles round her mouth, and in certain circumstances it can be harmful to the baby.

Before labour, therefore, we teach the woman what to expect and train her to relax. In labour we aim to keep her as calm as possible by giving her physical and emotional support, and by encouraging her to use what she has learned. To prevent hyperventilation we ask her to let her breathing remain quiet and as automatic as possible, and if it shows signs of becoming forced, or predominantly using the upper chest, to try to keep it 'low and slow'.

It is suggested that a woman should handle contractions in labour as follows: at the beginning she should ignore contractions, continuing normal activity as long as possible. If the contractions become painful and are causing symptoms of stress such as clenching the hands or jaws she should get into a position of ease, whether standing, sitting or lying. At the beginning of the contraction she should give a long easy breath out through a slightly rounded mouth in order to signal to her brain that she needs to concentrate on relaxing her whole body and prevent emphasis on the intake of breath. She should then close her lips and pause until her body is ready to breathe in at any depth or speed it chooses. She repeats this routine throughout each contraction. If the woman becomes distressed at the end of either the first or second stage of labour she should use an 'SOS' technique—that is, 'sigh out slowly', but still allow the breath to flow in through the nose when it is ready. She should understand that her breathing may change during different phases of labour and also from contraction to contraction depending on their length and strength, but should as far as possible 'tune in' to her body's needs so allowing the normal interchange of gases in the blood to proceed smoothly.

Breathing in the second stage of labour is based on the work of Caldeyro-Barcia (Stevenson, 1978). He found that if urged to block her breathing by closing her glottis and holding her breath, and straining as if constipated, there is initially a marked rise in blood pressure putting a strain on the muscles of the pelvic floor and abdominal wall, then a fall in blood pressure which is transmitted through the placenta and leads to hypoxia of the foetus. He, therefore, advocated that a mother should only push when she had the urge to do so and each effort should not last longer then 5–6 seconds.

At the John Radcliffe, maternal positions vary but frequently the mother is supported in an almost upright position with knees flexed and widely abducted, either with her hands on the outside of her knees and feet lifted off the bed when pushing or with the outer borders of her feet resting on the bed. When the urge to push is felt the mother is asked to drop her chin on her chest, and go with the contraction, strong breath holding is discouraged. After a few seconds she will want to pause, breathe in and repeat the manoeuvre. She tries to keep her legs and pelvic floor relaxed and can hiss gently to prevent pushing into her throat. It is important for the woman to realise that her body will guide her actions in the second stage providing her senses are not clouded by drugs.

The experimental work at John Radcliffe is continuing but the staff feel that these methods lead to calmer and less tired mothers and the babies are in better condition. Caldeyro-Barcia says that he has proved that his management of the second stage may lead to a longer stage then is sometimes considered desirable but the mothers are much less tired, there is less need for episiotomy and the Apgar score of the babies is better.

REFERENCES

Lum, L. (1975) Hyperventilation: The tip of the iceberg. *Journal of Psychosomatic Research*, **19**, 375–383.

Noble, E. (1981) Controversies in maternal effort during labour & delivery, *Journal of Nurse Midwifery* (U.S.A.), **26**, 2.

Stevenson, P. (1980) Report of address by Dr R. Caldeyro-Barcia, 1978, Maternal position and pushing during the second stage of labour. *Newsletter of The Association of Chartered Physiotherapists in Obstetrics and Gynaecology.*

FURTHER READING

Borning beds, Information from the Borning Corporation, 161, Adams, Spokane, Washington 99004.

Dale, B., Roeber, J. (1982) *Exercises for Childbirth*. London: Century Publishing Co.

Haddad, F. (1982) Alternative positions for labour. *Midwife, Health Visitor and Community Nurse*, **18**, 290–294.

Liu, Y. C. (1980) Effects of upright position during labour. *American Journal of Nursing*, 74, 2203–5.

Odent, M. (1980) Obstetric position, consciousness and maternity practice. *Journal of Biological Research*, 2, 9–14.

9

The puerperium and baby care

Families today are small and often widely scattered so that many young couples, unless they are lucky enough to live near friends who have a baby, rarely see or handle one. It is hardly surprising that they are unable to envisage their own baby or to picture what changes it will bring in their lives. They may have fantasies about the baby, the woman seeing it as the the smiling, active five-month-old baby of the milk food advertisements, while her husband may skip the whole babyhood phase and think of his son as a three-year-old child learning to kick a ball. Both these parents may be badly shaken when faced with the utterly helpless and infinitely demanding reality. If they have neither talked about nor seen pictures of newly-born babies they may be very shocked by the first appearance of their baby, its cord or afterbirth, and the exciting achievement of birth may be marred for them.

In spite of unreal fantasies and difficult deliveries many parents, particularly mothers, seem to have an immediate upsurge of love when they see their baby for the first time, which deepens as the days go by and they watch with fascination its first tentative efforts to explore its world. Other parents who have also embarked on pregnancy truly believing that it would deepen and enrich their lives, do not always fall immediately in love with their baby. These parents may feel disappointed and even guilty if their feelings do not match up to the lyrical descriptions in the books. Presumably because of the looser physical tie, some fathers only fall in love with their babies as they grow older and begin to communicate with them. At first these men may be jealous of their wife's involvement with the baby and what they see as a transfer of affection from themselves, particularly if the wife is breast feeding.

A few women who have become pregnant by mistake, or who have accepted pregnancy through some social pressure rather than a true desire for motherhood, may be worried by a lack of identification with the baby in *utero*. They may expect a great change in their feelings after the baby is born; some achieve this, but sadly in a few cases it never happens and these babies are never valued for themselves but only as some sort of symbol for their mothers. Thus, all parents need to be forewarned that having a baby is rather like having a love affair—sometimes strong and enduring feelings take time to develop.

All women fear for their children and some are actually afraid of them, often simply because they feel clumsy and inept over all these new tasks but sometimes for deep subconscious reasons of which they are not aware. An immature girl who is very dependent on her own mother may strive to please her baby in the way that she has tried to please her mother, and become frightened if her baby shows its 'disapproval' of her by crying or feeding poorly. Occasionally pregnancy reawakens memories of the births of brothers and sisters, the woman feels guilty about her dislike of her own mother in these situations and may transfer this guilt to her own baby, fearing that something will go wrong with it or herself as a punishment for these feelings. Parents who have themselves been brought up in an uncaring, unloving atmosphere find it much harder to love their babies, and in a few cases may dislike them so much that they actually cause them psychological or physical harm.

Multigravidae, particularly those who have one other young child, are often more concerned with the reactions of this child, so much so that they may wonder whether they are ever going to be able to love the new baby as much as the toddler. If they have had a bad first labour experience they may be very frightened of the second but at least they know that they are capable of giving birth, of recovering afterwards and of caring for a child, though they may wonder how they are going to make time for all the extra jobs.

Although most primigravidae say that the sex of their baby is immaterial as long as it is healthy, some women and, more particularly, men do have a great longing for a boy or girl and multigravidae usually hope for a child of different sex from the one they have. Disappointment usually fades quickly but an unfulfilled wish for a child of a particular sex may influence the handling of that child throughout its early years. Both parents like to see in their children characteristics they loved in their own parents or, if they have a good marriage relationship, in each other. Alternatively, they may be quick to censure in their children a trait that they dislike in themselves or in each other.

It is impossible to separate the mother's physical and emotional changes in the puerperium from her developing relationship with her baby, but an attempt must be made to prepare her for some of them since many women believe that as soon as their delivery is safely accomplished they will immediately regain their figures and become their prepregnancy selves again. They forget the tremendous physical, let alone emotional changes, which will take place in them and the stresses of life in hospital which to many are a completely new experience. Most children are jealous of a new baby and multigravidae need help in minimising and coping with the manifestations of this problem and in planning their daily activities to give adequate time to baby and toddler. When they go home or the midwife leaves, all women become easily tired and worried by the demands made upon them. After the first few weeks, when their absorption in the baby is beginning to wane, they may be torn between their new functions as a mother and the resumption of a job or other interests.

The following quotations from two letters may help to point out some of these changes. One mother wrote, 'Why had no one ever warned me that having a baby changes you unutterably? I had read thousands of words on how to care for babies, how to help them reach their potential, how to clean their bottoms and mix their feeds, but I hadn't read anything which significantly impressed on me that having a baby would work a major change on my life and on my life style. I didn't understand that she would cause an upheaval, this '8 lb volcano' at once so helpless and so fiercely demanding, that she would transform our lives and rearrange them.' Another mother said, 'Having a baby puts you into an older age group—your friends, your conversation and your priorities change. I'm already aware that I'm in the next generation, there's an enormous gulf which separates you from being young and in love from being parents and in love.'

How then can we help men and women to set out on this very long voyage of parenthood? How many attitudes must we accept as already formed during childhood, schooldays or love affairs? How much must be left until after the baby is born? Can we do anything during pregnancy to modify unhelpful attitudes and to prepare the parents-to-be or their other children?

We can certainly be aware of some of the psychological factors underlying the changes from 'people in love' to 'parents in love' and discuss changes in life style with the group. We can help these young people a little way along their road to maturity by minimising our authoritarian teaching and persuading them to think for themselves about many aspects of their new undertaking, whether this be planning the baby's layette, coping with it when it cries, dealing with a jealous toddler or future family planning. Throughout these sessions we can reassure them that although outside help will be available they will quickly come to know their own baby's needs and their own instincts will usually guide them in satisfying these.

We can make sure that new mothers do know what a young baby looks like and what it can do. It should be possible for each member of the group who has not done so before, to hold a small baby. Mothers calling into class at coffee time to talk of their experiences are delighted to have one or two of the group holding and admiring their babies while they talk, or during a visit to the maternity unit permission may be sought for somebody to pick up one of the babies who is not asleep.

We should certainly not neglect practical advice, but keep it short and simple, stressing the broad principles of feeding, cleaning and communicating rather than unimportant details such as which arm is washed first. All this teaching will be repeated after the baby is born whether in hospital or at home. Some midwives report that the mothers retain a lot of class teaching, others that the immediacy of having to cope with their babies is the only stimulus to learning baby care. Whether the class member retains much of the content or not, however, it appears to add to her sense of preparedness of 'becoming a mother', if she has participated in classes on bathing, feeding and handling a baby during her pregnancy.

A talk on the third stage of labour leads simply into the early, then later changes of the puerperium from the mother's, then father's, point of view. It is easy to make the early changes sound like just a list of discomforts from sore tails, afterpains, engorged breasts to postpartum blues, but possible to stress also the positive joys of returning quickly to full health while watching the first fascinating days of the baby's development. We can end with a discussion on the resumption of intercourse, future family planning and the value of the postnatal check.

Finally, and perhaps most important of all, by the way every member of the staff talks to the group, by the illustrations we select and the films we show, we can convey something, not only of the 'problems of parenthood', but of its joys and our acceptance of its tremendous social value to the community.

PLANNING BABY-CARE INSTRUCTION

As was said in Chapter 1, the major aim of many women who come to antenatal classes is to seek help in understanding and coping with labour. Planning of the baby's layette and equipment must be done early in the course or preferably soon after booking, perhaps at an evening meeting to which both parents are invited. But the amount of further information on baby-care that even an intelligent primigravida can take in seems to be very limited and will often only be accepted after the more immediate problems of labour have been fully discussed. As a woman becomes increasingly clumsy and uncomfortable at the end of pregnancy, she longs, on one hand, to be free of her burden but, on the other, may fear the separation from her child and all the new responsibilities she will have in caring for it outside her womb. We find that it is during these last few weeks that information and discussion on baby-care is eagerly accepted. We must presume a certain amount of inattention, and so put emphasis on important points, making the teaching as vivid and varied as possible, an onslaught on the eyes, ears and, if possible, hands.

A suggested syllabus follows.

Early in pregnancy

Planning the baby's room and surroundings. Safety precautions. Clothes. Equipment—buying the minimum and choosing with care to fit parents' way of life, mother's height, etc. Preparing other children for the birth of the baby.

Breast changes during pregnancy. Hygiene—discussion and demonstration of suitable bras, how to put them on and when to wear them. Exercises for muscles of the chest wall underlying the breasts. Discussion of pros and cons of breast feeding. For those who may want to breast feed: care of the nipples, possibility of wearing Waller shells, demonstration of hand positions for expression of colostrum if teacher is in favour of this manoeuvre.

Later in pregnancy (after labour classes)

Bathing—preferably a demonstration on a real baby or, failing this, an attractive life-size doll handled by the teacher with the tenderness she would use for a baby.

Breast feeding Reassurance that the vast majority of women can breast feed if they really want to. Advantages of putting the baby to the breast soon after delivery, seeking cooperation of the lactation Sisters, when available. The production of milk and the let-down reflex—how these are influenced by glands and emotions. Getting baby on and off the breast, checking its sucking, winding it.

Pleasurable sensations—early difficulties and how to treat them. Books and leaflets for those who want to know more.

Bottle feeding. Method of suppressing lactation in local units—some discomfort likely. Demonstration and discussion of different types of bottles and teats, allowing mothers to handle these. Sterilisation of equipment and its importance. Mixing feeds of different types. Clearing away and washing up. Advice on husband and wife practising routine beforehand with their own equipment so that all can be ready for the baby's first feed at home. Points about holding and handling the baby to simulate breast feeding as far as possible. Demand feeding.

The baby's appearance and activities.

The puerperium. Hospital routine. Physical and emotional changes in the mother. Postnatal exercises. The beginning of the parents' relationship with their baby and his care.

Special care nurseries (see p. 193).

Parenthood. Fitting the baby into the home environment with husband, siblings, grandparents. Further physical and emotional changes in the mother including fatigue, with ideas on its prevention. Mother's occasional ambivalence between love of her baby and re-establishment both of her own ego and her life with her husband. Resumption of intercourse, family planning. Postnatal check, cervical cytology. Further development of the baby.

PRESENTATION AND EXPLANATIONS

Planning for the baby

This could simply be a talk, but our teaching requirements of 'an onslaught on the eyes, ears and hands' call for a different approach.

We can begin by describing the preparation and effective heating of the baby's room and start a discussion on the merits of putting him straight into it, or of sharing with parents or other children. Continue by making points about choosing a cot, carrycot and pram to suit each family's way of life, illustrated by cut-outs from advertisements and baby magazines. Suggest economy measures, such as cutting down a kitchen chair to make a nursing chair, covering a cardboard box with gay plastic material instead of buying an expensive toilet basket, or using the kitchen sink instead of a small bath. One of us uses a good photograph of one of her daughters at the age of five months being bathed in a caravan sink to illustrate this point.

A modern layette can then be produced with alternatives, such as babygros and nightdresses, differently shaped vests, cardigans with buttons or bows, nylon and cotton dresses, shaped and plain napkins of different sizes and textures, various styles of plastic pants and disposable napkins. To involve the group in activity they can be asked to choose the clothes they would buy, and how many of each article they would need. A chalk board and chalk is then necessary. The class can be divided into groups of convenient size (perhaps two groups of six to eight members) with one member appointed as 'reporter'. The layette is left with the groups for 10 minutes, and in this time the teacher writes on the board the articles of clothing, with three columns, one for each group and one for herself. The groups decide what they would buy, and the quantity. These are written in the appropriate columns, and the teacher adds her own choice, explaining her reasons as she does so (for example, a winter baby is warmer in an envelope-type vest and a babygro than in a vest with tie fastening and a nightdress). Points where the groups differ from each other and from the teacher usually provide lots of conversation and any multigravida in the class can add practical points from her own experience.

Breast and bottle feeding

A discussion on methods of feeding a young baby raises a number of problems for the teacher since she is likely to have strong personal prejudices in favour of using breast or bottle. These may arise from her professional knowledge and observation or more subtly from her personal experience of the joys or disappointments associated with feeding her own babies.

A mother's decision whether or not to nurse her baby, as with her reactions to pregnancy and labour, is not an isolated one; it depends on many factors, such as her upbringing, her feeling about her body, her husband's views and the climate of opinion in her peer group. Public opinion about baby feeding is at present in the process of interesting changes in different parts of the world. In this country before the Industrial Revolution, mother's milk was the accepted food for a baby and it was a stigma if one was not able to produce enough. This gradually changed with the employment of women outside the home and the mass production of a satisfactory container—the glass bottle. Early in the century the mortality of artificially fed babies was four to six times greater than breast fed babies, but with the improvement of hygiene and sanitation bottle feeding became relatively safe. Women began to accept it as the norm and to regard breast feeding as somewhat 'low class and primitive', an attitude which is prevalent in many developing countries today. The rejection of the primary function of the female breasts reached its height in the United States where breasts became a major sex symbol for enjoyment by husbands not babies.

During the last few years in this country there has been a marked swing back towards breast feeding, at least during the early weeks of a baby's life (Page, 1971). This originated with the better educated mothers, particularly in Social Classes I and II, from their reading and discussions on the physical and emotional benefits to their babies and themselves, and appears to be spreading to other groups. The discovery of the increased risk of thrombo-embolism among mothers when lactation is suppressed by oestrogens has led to the abandonment of these drugs for this purpose. The return to older methods of suppressing lactation, which sometimes give rise to considerable discomfort, may also be a contributory factor in promoting breast feeding. Since this book was first written the swing has become more marked among all sections of the population. Today if one asks a class of mothers-to-be how they plan to feed their babies only two or three out of a group of 20–30 will opt for bottle feeding. In spite of their wishes, regrettably many do not succeed, as was shown by a survey reported in the *Nursing Times* in 1977. It was found that less than 30% of a large sample of mothers were breast feeding at one month and only 6% at three months. It was, however, reported that in areas where doctors and midwives gave active support 20% of the mothers were still breast feeding at three months.

It is interesting to consider why so many mothers now wish to breast feed and why so many later give up. There has recently been a great deal of publicity both in professional and lay circles about the value of breast feeding, much of it based on the authoritative report by the Department of Health and Social Security working party under the chairmanship of Professor T. Oppé entitled 'Present-day practice in infant feeding'. This states that the members of the working party are convinced that 'when successfully managed, breast feeding of 4–6 months duration offers many advantages to both mother and infant, and effectively safeguards the infant from the adverse conditions which are, or may be, associated with artificial feeding. Since the risks of ill health are greater when the baby is very young breast feeding for even as short a period as two weeks is an advantage'.

Recently a number of new books and films have been produced, some of which are listed at the end of this chapter and in the film section. The subject is being openly discussed in schools and clubs along with many other aspects of sexuality. It seems that a large proportion of today's primiparae want the experience for their babies and themselves, but we have not yet reached the stage when all of them are given adequate help.

Professional attitudes are also in a state of flux. At first many midwives and doctors tried to stem the flood of demand for bottle feeding and some went so far as to insist that *all* the mothers in their care should attempt to breast feed. Psychiatrists pointed out that an unwilling mother is not likely to succeed, would feel guilty about her failure and the resulting situation might well do real harm to her relationship with her baby. The opinions of many professionals then changed, particularly those of the younger hospital workers and they themselves began to feel guilty if they over-persuaded a reluctant mother. Some midwives preferred regular artificial feeding using presterilised bottles as a quick way out for themselves. In some units, although lip service is paid to the practices of rooming-in and demand feeding, some mothers have still to fight for the privilege of putting the baby to the breast in the labour ward, and being allowed to feed the baby at frequent intervals, particularly during the night. The use of water in between feeds and refusal to give cow's milk at any time except in special circumstances is still not universal practice; nor is time and support in a calm atmosphere to establish lactation, particularly after a difficult delivery. Some hospitals have appointed a member of staff whose special duty is to supervise the preparation for and practice of all forms of infant feeding and these Sisters have been found to be of great value since they are relieved of other midwifery duties and have more time to spend with the mothers. Voluntary associations such as the Breast Feeding Promotion Group of the National Childbirth Trust, the La Leche League and the Nursing Mothers' Association of Australia still find that they have plenty to do in designing propaganda for professionals, in educating parents and in supporting them when the mothers come home.

When planning classes on infant feeding we must first of all get our facts straight, separating those which have a good experimental basis from those which can be traced to wishful thinking on the part of the enthusiasts for one or other method. For example, there is now plenty of evidence to show that the chemical composition of human milk is more suitable for a baby's digestion than cow's milk however modified.

S. J. Darke (1975) Principal Medical Officer for Nutrition to the

DHSS notes that the higher concentration of protein in undiluted cow's milk can be associated with an increase in blood urea. It may also predispose to such allergic diseases as asthma and eczema. The higher blood concentration of amino-acids may also not be without harm, in that neurological sequelae have been reported in premature and full-term low birth weight infants. Some claims have been made that the difference in fatty acid patterns of human and cow's milk may be important in the development of the lipids of the central nervous system. The higher concentration in cow's milk of inorganic nutrients such as calcium and phosphorus may be a factor in the aetiology of neonatal tetany. The higher sodium ion content may also be harmful to a baby's kidneys particularly in conditions which lead to an excessive loss of fluid through the skin.

It has long been known that breast fed babies are much less prone to infection than bottle fed babies, especially in surroundings where hygiene is poor. Until recently this protection was thought to be largely passive, that is to say that human milk is less likely to be contaminated than the prepared bottle feed. Recently there has been much new information to show that the soluble whey of human milk contain species specific proteins which have built-in anti-infective properties. There seems little doubt that overweight babies lead to overweight adults with the attendant disadvantages (Creery, 1973) and the risk of a too rapid gain of weight is more common when a too large or too concentrated cow's milk formula is given or solids, particularly carbohydrates, are introduced too early.

The physical effects of breast feeding on the mother, namely a quicker involution of the uterus and a suppression or diminution of ovulation, are widely accepted. At an international conference on the epidemiology of cancer held in Yugoslavia in 1972, it was reported that the tendency to mammary cancer was markedly diminished only in women whose first lactation was early in life.

The psychological effects of breast feeding both on the mother and her baby, though frequently discussed, are very difficult to prove. Evidence is accumulating that frequent contact between mother and baby very soon after birth and at more frequent intervals than those required simply for feeding has a beneficial effect on the mother-child relationship, and that these children begin to communicate at an earlier age (Klaus et al., 1972). Contact, particularly of skin to skin, is much more natural in the breast feeding situation, though its non-acceptance may be at the root of a decision to bottle feed, but if the value of handling, touching and talking to her baby is pointed out to the bottle-feeding mother there seems no reason why she and her baby should not get many of the benefits of being together.

However, more recent research (Whittlestone, 1977) suggests that the act of suckling causes a release of both prolactin and oxytocin in a normal woman, but the opportunity only to play with her baby, while releasing oxytocin, does *not* release prolactin. This means that in the case of the mother bottle feeding her child, unless she has established a very strong prolactin reflex following an initial breast feeding period she may not continue to release prolactin so that the mother—baby bond will tend to weaken.

Thus there seems to be overwhelming evidence that there are important benefits of breast feeding to both baby and mother. It must be remembered though, that it is estimated that about 10% of women are unable to feed their babies for various reasons and there will always be others who either have to go back to work or who prefer to use cow's milk. It may be a stigma on our way of life but it is certainly true that some women simply cannot believe that their bodies will be adequate for their new task. Especially if there are some early set-backs they will not persevere, and will opt for a bottle where they can see exactly how much their baby has taken. Wise handling during the puerperium may overcome these difficulties but it is fatally easy for the unenthusiastic doctor or midwife to take the easy way out. We must therefore not allow a mother who wishes to bottle feed to feel guilty, or that she has failed, and must help her to choose a suitable modified milk and to prepare and use it skilfully.

We have heard a number of women who have successfully fed a first baby, saying that they are thinking of giving the new baby the bottle because it will be easier to manage the toddler at the same time and give rise to less jealousy. As with so many other aspects of the coming baby, a little child needs to be prepared beforehand. He must have a simple explanation of the way the new baby will get his milk, demonstrated if possible by a friend's baby or animal or even animal pictures and will then usually accept suckling as quite common-place, providing it is made clear that the baby is drinking milk that comes *out* of the mother's body not that the baby is *eating* her and that he also, as a baby, drank in this way. When the time comes he will like to have a book read to him or special toys to play with during the feed when he is present (wise planning will often reduce this to one or two sessions a day). He is likely to want to play at being a baby himself and if allowed to suckle for a few minutes, will quickly decide that a cup is easier for him. Small boys and girls alike will want to play at being mother and will try to nurse dolls and teddies and get cross when no milk is produced. Normal jealousies that are aroused then seem to come from the family changes rather than from the breast feeding situation and are minimal if wisely handled.

Bearing some of these points in mind, how then can we encourage those who are sure that they wish to nurse their babies, influence those who are doubtful, yet still help those who are convinced that bottle feeding is right for them? We might perhaps start by pointing out to the class that a baby's earliest pleasure comes from feeding, and if the mother also derives pleasure from this activity it will give her a tremendous sense of her personal value and importance to her baby and it is likely that a firm emotional closeness will quickly build up between them. On the other hand, if a woman nurses only because she considers it her duty and derives no satisfaction from the process, she is unlikely to make either her baby or herself happy. Most new mothers will have little idea whether or not they are going to enjoy nursing and it is surely our duty to persuade them to keep an open mind and to enthuse them enough for them to have a try. If members of the group come from families where breast feeding is not customary, they may never even have seen a baby at the breast. It is usually easy to rectify this situation by introducing the group to a mother in one of the lying-in wards who is breast feeding or by inviting one to visit the class with her baby. We may, in addition, bring in a bottle-feeding mother and sit back while the group talk. If mothers and babies are unavailable, a film (see film list) may be a useful way of starting a group discussion and can also be used at a fathers' evening. We can sum up by presenting the pros and cons as honestly and unemotionally as we are able, and this together with a short talk on breast changes and care would make a good introductory class. This might be followed later in the course by two further classes of practical hints on breast and bottle feeding.

We should never minimise the problems of breast feeding, to quote E. Tylden (1975) 'Breast feeding is not instinctive. Successful breast feeding is only attained through practice, it cannot be learned by watching, though this helps. Nor can it be learned by reading books any more than can typing or playing the piano'. It is not uncommon even among animals for females to lose their first young through failure to manage their feeding. Therefore although we can set the scene during pregnancy the drama takes place in the lying-in wards and is only finished when feeding patterns are finally established at home in the family setting.

The baby's appearance and activities

There are many publications which describe new babies, ranging from text books of paediatrics to baby food advertisements; each teacher will pick from them the answers to the questions she is commonly asked. Many mothers seem to have found the following points helpful.

'Some months ago we listened to a psychiatrist giving a vivid description of what he felt like when he was born and claiming that it is possible to uncover memories of birth in other people and the influence these memories have had on their lives. Be that as it may, birth must be a tremendous shock for a baby. He has lived for nine months in a warm, moist, dark world, listened to the comforting beat of his mother's heart, and been supplied with food and oxygen without any effort. He may have been disturbed occasionally by some movement of his mother's body and wriggled himself into a more comfortable position or been startled by some sudden noise, but basically he has had a very peaceful, protected life.

'During birth all this changes: he is subjected to tremendous pressures as the contractions of the womb mount in intensity, twisted, turned, and squeezed through a narrow canal and finally ejected into a cold, bright, noisy world. He has to learn to eat and breathe and gradually come to accept that he is no longer part of his mother. It is hardly surprising that it takes him a few days, a few weeks or even a few months to settle down to this new existence. We can help him along the path by the way we handle him, but each baby, like each adult, will go his own pace in his own way.

'When you get a chance to have a real look at your baby you'll find his head looks rather big for his body, the forehead flattened and the back elongated, due to pressure during birth. You'll notice two soft spots or fontanelles on his skull where the bones have not yet joined, you can often see a pulse beating through the larger one close to the front of the crown of his head. Don't believe tales that you mustn't touch a baby's head because of these soft spots, for the brain is covered by a very tough membrane, although it is not yet completely bone. His face may disappoint you, unless you expect to see pudgy cheeks, a broad flat nose and an undersized lower jaw, though the fact that he is wrinkled and toothless may give him an uncanny look of one of his grandparents.

'His eyes usually look dark blue and have a blank staring gaze, and he may seem to squint because he has not yet learned to focus. Although his world is a blur he can distinguish between light and darkness but prefers the latter as he is more used to it. His eyelids may be rather puffy.

'His limbs may seem rather puny and undeveloped and his legs tend to be drawn up towards his tummy in their pre-birth position. His abdomen will look rounded and have a stump of the cord, now an empty tube of skin under a light dressing. Genitals, particularly of boy babies, tend to look large compared with the rest of the body. Two or three days after birth you may be surprised to find that a girl baby occasionally has a tiny false menstrual period, while babies of both sexes may produce a little milk in their breasts. These changes are due to adjustments in the mother's body chemistry at the end of pregnancy and quickly fade. All babies lose weight during the first few days of life due to loss of body fluids; they are given boiled water, sometimes with glucose, to counteract this, before the mother's milk comes in.

'A baby's skin is thin and dry and may be somewhat blotchy. A deep flush spreads over his entire body if he cries hard and the veins of his head may swell but you will notice no tears as the tear ducts do not function yet. If he is deeply asleep his body loses colour and looks pale and his hands and feet soon become cold if he is not well wrapped up. A few days after birth he may look slightly yellowish because he is getting rid of the extra blood cells in which he has been storing oxygen while inside you. He now no longer needs this because he is breathing oxygen from the air.

Jaundice

'Some years ago, babies used to be born from Rh-positive mothers with a definite yellow skin colour. This does not happen now, but 'physiological jaundice' is being watched more seriously. What happens is that at about two or three days old, the baby looks as if he has come from the South of France, and obtained a golden tan. The difficulty is that, when inside you, he had to have lots of red blood cells to absorb the oxygen you were giving him. When breathing his own oxygen, he has too many red blood cells, and the liver has to absorb them. If the liver is slow to do this, jaundice occurs, and the baby looks beautifully healthy but is sleepy. Today, blood is taken from all yellowish babies to see how the absorption is going on. If it is slow, the baby is given phototherapy. This word worries mothers, but it simply means that the baby is placed, for part of the day, naked under fluorescent lights. He is very warm, and the mother is encouraged to handle and stroke him. The only thing which may be worrying is that his eyes will be covered to protect them from the light. This doesn't bother him—he has been in the dark for nine months—but makes a mother sometimes feel very protective and distressed. If this happens, be with your baby, talk to him, hold him—you will feel better. Expect him to be rather sleepy still when the phototherapy is finished—make the most of the peace! He doesn't really need extra fluids, but the heat of the lamp makes it necessary that, even though sleepy, he has adequate feeds. (Some hospitals give extra water, but this is often refused by the sleepy baby.)

Other conditions

'Several tests have been developed to give the baby a good start in life. One is the "Guthrie" test, a tiny spot of blood from a heel prick at a few days of age. This shows that he is not the one in 10 000 who have phenylketonuria (a genetic defect) but if he happens to be the one, he can immediately be identified and have a special diet, which includes a little milk, but mostly a specially prepared formula low in the amino-acid phenylalanine. One of us has recently cared for an infant who, surprisingly perhaps, much preferred the formula to the milk. He has developed into an extremely bright, active toddler. If this test had not been carried out, he would have had brain damage before he was a year old. Another test is from the cord blood—to see if the mother has Rh antigens in her bloodstream (see p. 93). A third is from the first stool passed—the dark meconium— which can identify fibrocystic disease and any baby with this rare condition can have early treatment.'

Special care nurseries

'Special care nurseries used to be reserved for premature and small-for-dates babies and babies who had experienced difficult deliveries. The latter still applies to some extent, but premature, healthy babies are allowed to be with their mothers. "Special care" is mostly appropriate to babies with breathing difficulties—"Respiratory Distress Syndrome" (RDS) meaning that their lungs did not function well from birth. Oxygen, and injections to develop their lungs, are given, and the results are good. Mothers are encouraged to come into the unit, and even if baby is in an incubator, to stroke and hold him, so that contact is not broken in the few days after birth when both mother and child require the touch and feel of each other ("bonding" is the "in" word) but the child can experience love, and, in the mother, love grows. Very small babies are, of course, still given this 'special care'.

Compared with many animal babies such as foals and calves which must be able to stagger after their mothers a few hours after birth, a human baby may seem incredibly ill-equipped to face the world but he has some skills which will help him to survive. If his face is touched he will turn his head to that side, and a touch on his lips with nipple or finger encourages him to open his mouth and begin to suck anything that is put inside it, and if this is fluid he will swallow it. The most sensitive part of his whole body is his mouth and he gets great pleasure from using it, but do not assume that if he manages to get a finger or a bit of blanket into his mouth he is necessarily hungry—the sucking just makes him feel good.

'He can move freely but cannot yet control any single limb, so that when he cries his whole body jerks and moves. Some babies can lift their heads a little way off the mattress but none of them can hold their heads steady when they are in the upright position, so that their heads feel loose and must always be supported. When very young, they miss the confinement of the womb and like to be held firmly against the mother's body or to be fairly tightly wrapped in a blanket or shawl. They have an inborn fear of being dropped, hence will sometimes quieten when cuddled by an experienced midwife or grandmother instead of being rather gingerly handled by an inexperienced mother. Later on they love to be free of all clothes and kick on a rug in the sunlight or swim and swish in the bath.

'A baby has one endearing habit which can be made use of when introducing him to another child: he will grasp and cling to any object such as a finger which is put into the palm of his hand. This is said to be the remnant of our monkey ancestry when we had to cling to our mother's fur as she swung through the trees. However we don't need to tell the toddler this and he thinks that *his* baby is holding *his* hand.

'Babies do not mind a certain amount of noise having been used to the noises inside and outside their mother's bodies, but they are apt to wake and cry if the noise level suddenly changes—an aeroplane passes overhead or the telephone rings. They love to be talked to and sung to (you don't have to keep in tune!) and quickly respond to the tone of a person's voice long before words have any meaning for them. also they will learn to smile back if their mother smiles at them—their first "social" response.

'A baby has only one way of telling you that he is unhappy and that is to cry. Some authorities claim that mothers learn to differentiate between cries for help of different kinds, such as food, pain or attention. We have not found this to be true; the crying of a healthy baby certainly varies in intensity from intermittent grizzling to a full-throated yell but it seems to be only through experience and trial and error that the particular need can be satisfied. In a recent American survey of 80 healthy babies whose mothers were encouraged to give them every care, on an average a six-week-old baby cried for two hours and 45 minutes each day. At 10 weeks the crying began to taper off and by three months the average was one hour. The author concluded that some babies cry for exercise and the fun of hearing their own voices, in the same way that some women chatter aimlessly. Even with this comforting thought, most women find it very worrying when their babies go on crying but should remember to check the obvious things first, like hunger, wind, the need for a change of position or clothing or often the need for company, and a cuddle, before deciding that the baby is ill or they are bad mothers. Perhaps too many of us expect the baby to lie still, when he has been bounced around inside us for so many months. A sling, such as an "Easy-Rider", could give him the movements that he needs to soothe him.

'Some babies undoubtedly enjoy wetting or soiling themselves and only protest if they become sore or cold, others do not like the feel of a dirty nappy; mothers are often much more sensitive than their babies on this point. The first stools are blackish green, then they become bright mustard yellow, but breast-fed babies may only pass a motion every two or three days.

'Remember that a baby's greatest pleasures are suckling, being touched and rocked or patted rhythmically, so that feeding times are enormously important. He needs time to suck, to rest and suck again, to touch, feel and smell his mother's breast if she is nursing him, her hands and face if she is not, to listen to her voice, watch her smile and feel the comfort of her arms as she pats him gently on the back.'

The puerperium

Some suggestions for describing a newly born baby have already been given; it is also hoped that parents will be able to see pictures and movies of new babies or better still to look at and hold a young baby before their own labour experience. It is important that the antenatal teacher should be familiar with the routine in the lying-in wards of her local hospitals or the nursing care given by her local midwives. She can then describe briefly the outline of a typical day during the early puerperium and answer queries on points such as 'How soon will my baby be allowed to stay with me?', or 'When can I get up?

A talk on the mother's reactions may usefully be introduced by asking members of the group to describe their own, following a previous confinement, or those of friends and relations. Two sharply contrasting patterns of behaviour often emerge from this discussion, one characterised by intense excitement and fulfilment, the other a rather passive relief at the end of an ordeal. Continue thus:

'After a hard labour, particularly if you have needed a lot of medication, you may indeed be weary and disinterested in your baby, wanting only to relax and sleep, but even if you have had a tough time you may, on the other hand, be on top of the world, hungry and active and need an unwinding period before you can rest. If your husband has not been present you may want to go through your labour, telling him all the good and the bad bits and possibly to work off some resentment either with your own behaviour or that of the staff.

'You may just be happy to know that your baby is safe, healthy and well cared for or you may have an intense longing to see and touch him. You may know quite well that the hospital rules say that your baby must be kept in the nursery for a certain length of time, yet have a nagging doubt that "they" are doing it because there is "something wrong".

Although you have been longing to be yourself again you may be surprised how empty your body now feels and that you miss the companionship of the baby's movements. At first you may be a bit put off by the appearance of your tummy being "rather like cheap seersucker" as one mother descibed it to me recently. You will all be longing to get your figures back and if you have done your exercises during pregnancy, go on working hard at them afterwards and watch your diet, I can promise that you will succeed. We will practise a few easy exercises in a moment.

'Your tail may feel bruised or sore if you have had stitches or the lower part of your body may feel numb, so much so that you may be unaware for a long time of a need to pass water. You will have a blood-stained discharge, heavier than a normal period, and may pass a few small clots; these are usually nothing to worry about but the midwives will be keeping an eye on them. They will also check your pulse, temperature and blood pressure at intervals and measure the position of the top part of your uterus to make sure that it is gradually going down. This involution or shrinking of the uterus is achieved by further contractions of its muscles so you haven't finished with these when your baby is born. You will often feel these contractions at the time that you are feeding your baby because the same hormone that stimulates milk production also stimulates the uterus. They usually pass quickly if you relax and concentrate on breathing through them, but sometimes they do merit the description of after-pains and Sister may give you something to help.

'During the next few days you'll have the thrill of getting to know your baby, watching his movements, listening to the different noises that he makes and the way he reacts to your touch and care. It's comforting to know that there is always skilled help to turn to, though in hospital you may get some conflicting advice—in this case the only course is to decide which member of the staff has ideas which you particularly like and which fit the way you feel about your baby and listen mainly to her. If it is your first baby, you will feel very incompetent and hopelessly ham-handed to start with, as baby-care, like any other skill, takes a while to acquire; but by the end of a week you'll be giving the new mothers tips. Some people enjoy the companionship and support of other mothers in a ward, others find the atmosphere too reminiscent of school or camp. Recently delivered women do undoubtedly behave rather like adolescent girls, their emotions are very near the surface and one moment they are giggling helplessly, while the next they may be in bitter tears over some real or imagined problem. You may find you are particularly sensitive and on edge two or three days after your baby is born: this is due partly to the big chemical changes which are taking place in your body as your milk begins to come in, partly to physical discomforts in breasts or tail, and partly a reaction to the big effort of labour and the dawning realisation of your new role and responsibilities. If you suddenly burst into tears or get annoyed with one of the midwives don't feel guilty about it, they will understand, but do remember that they are also women and have problems and emotions too. Above all, if you suddenly feel cross with your baby, don't immediately assume that you are totally unfitted for motherhood but merely that you need a good sleep or somebody understanding to talk to. It's a good idea to warn your husband about these possible ups and downs so that he will understand why you feel like this.

'Adequate rest in hospital is a problem, particularly if you are in a ward with other people and their babies. Even if you are alone, there is a great tendency to go calling or to be continually jumping in and out of bed. Do try to get all the sleep you can and observe any rules about rest periods or limitation of the number of visitors. Anyone who is having her baby as a private patient, where visiting may be almost unrestricted, needs to take this advice particularly to heart. Perhaps your husband could ask some of the relations to wait awhile; if visitors become overwhelming he may ask the doctor if visiting can be restricted for a while, and inform friends of the "doctor's" decision. He may like to suggest that fruit would be more acceptable than too many flowers or sweets.

'If it is not your first baby and child visitors are allowed do let the other children come to see you and the baby, even if they do not like leaving you behind. Psychiatrists agree that it is better for a two-year-old to cry at leaving mummy than not to see her and feel deserted. If children are not allowed to visit, you may be able to telephone home each day and can certainly take in a series of post-cards or little toys, one of which your husband can take home each evening to show your other child that your are thinking about him.'

The film strip 'More Tiny Feet' may be useful to show to multi-gravidae to help them both in preparing a toddler for a new baby and managing the toddler later. Another strip 'Your First Baby', Part 3, 'Afterwards', may also be useful in promoting discussion about some of the changes in the puerperium; it could be used instead of a talk with expansion on the points which the teacher felt to be particularly important. The recent film, 'With a little help' arouses interest in both primigravidae and multigravidae, and is excellent in its protrayal of the early days of parenthood.

Postnatal exercises

If it is known that a physiotherapist will be available to teach these exercises where the mothers in the group are being delivered, little need be said about them other than to impress their importance on the group. If, on the other hand, this is doubtful, it is very easy to explain how the antenatal exercises can be modified for use after delivery. Here are some ideas for a brief talk.

'There is nothing difficult about these exercises except the will-power to persevere with them, particularly after you go home, as it is fatally easy to say, "I'm tired tonight so I'll do them tomorrow." There will often be a physiotherapist to help you but, if not, you may need to get started by yourself. Check with you midwife that all is well, then you can begin as soon as you have had a few hours' rest after your baby is born. Take a few deep breaths in and out, trying to make the air go right down to the bottom of your lungs, expanding your chest much more deeply than you have been able to do for the last few months.

'Move your feet up and down and draw circles in the air with your big toes. Bend and stretch your knees, pressing your legs down hard on the bed. Lie on your back with both knees bent, feet flat on the bed, and try to pull your tummy in towards your backbone, just as you did when you were pregnant. Try each movement about four times then have a rest. Do the exercises four times a day—it is helpful to tie them with some other activity, say just before each meal, or just after you feed your baby, then you are less likely to forget.

'When you are told that you can get up to go to the toilet, don't wait till the last moment then make a dash—a lot of changes have been going on in your circulation and you may feel odd if you stand up in a hurry. Sit on the side of your bed and swing your legs for a few minutes, stand up slowly, pull your tummy in and brace your undercarriage, then move off. This routine was suggested by Eileen Montgomery in her book *At Your Best for Birth and Later* and has been found very useful.

'Twenty-four hours after you have had your baby you will find that you can pull your tummy in more strongly and can begin to flatten your back at the same time, thus "rocking your pelvis" as you have been used to doing. During pregnancy you did a gentle pull in and release of the muscles, but now you can tighten and tighten your tummy until it won't become even half an inch flatter, hold it while you count four, then relax.

'You can also begin to contract your pelvic floor muscles again, at first just trying to pull the whole muscle sling up, then gradually trying to separate off the back from the front passages. Remember that now we are trying to strengthen the muscles so the contraction needs to be held for a count of up to 10 before letting go slowly. You may find that the muscles feel numb and hard to control at first or, alternatively, that the contractions pull on your stitches. Persevere gently because the movement of the muscles and skin improves the blood flow and so helps to diminish swelling. Try frequently to stop the stream when you are passing urine, you should succeed in doing this a week to ten days after your baby's birth.

'When it is time for a rest, turn on your front, arranging two pillows under your tummy and two under your head, so that there is no pressure on your breasts. It will feel good to be off your tail. If you tighten your buttocks hard and relax them about six times, you will begin to strengthen the joints at the bottom of your spine which you will remember tend to slacken during pregnancy and labour and cause backache if they do not return to normal quickly. If any exercise or movement that you do gives you backache, be sure to stop for a few days before you try again.

When you sit up in bed or in a chair try to sit as upright as possible with the whole of your back supported; a pillow wedged into the small of your back may help. When you are feeding your baby, make sure that both of you are comfortable; if you have a long back you may be happier if he is resting on one or two pillows, particularly if you are breast feeding, so that he can easily reach your nipple without your having to stoop.' The teacher can demonstrate with pillows and a doll. 'When you stand or lift remember all the points we have made during the classes and that you will now have to adapt your balance once more to your changed weight.' The teacher recapitulates using examples applicable to the new situation, i.e. putting a baby into a cot or lifting a nappy bucket.

'You stop doing the breathing and foot exercises after the first two days unless otherwise instructed, but go on with the tummy, pelvic floor and buttock contractions four times a day for at least six weeks, increasing the number of contractions to eight for the tummy and buttocks but keeping the pelvic floor to four each time. After you are up and about again all day there is no need to lie down to do your exercises, as they can all be done while sitting or standing. The important thing is that they *are* done.'

If the teacher knows that competent supervision will be available no further instructions are necessary; if not, she may like to demonstrate some more advanced exercises herself or suggest one of the books at the end of this chapter. *You After Childbirth* and *Essential Exercises for the Childbearing Year* are excellent new books.

The problems of being a parent

This last session is conducted as a group discussion. It fits well into the latter part of a fathers' evening, so giving both parents the opportunity to think and talk about issues which are of such vital importance to them both, or discuss thoughts that may be arising now they are coming so close to producing this baby. If it is held for mothers only, then multigravidae, who often do not attend all the parentcraft sessions, should be encouraged to stay for this one because their contributions from experience are invaluable.

Discussion could be triggered off by showing a film, such as 'Their First Year', or a film strip (see Appendix for details). If there are several multigravidae in the group, the strip 'More Tiny Feet' may be appreciated. Alternatively, points from letters could be read, or a quotation from a book, such as the following: 'Take as many cat-naps as you can fit in during the day while the baby sleeps. You're going to need them in the first few weeks. Some days may go like a dream. Others may seem hellish. You're cross with your husband. You can't stand his mother's advice. You're overtired. You hate the baby. It seems to cry non-stop. You're overwhelmed and feel you can't cope' (Fae Winn, in *New Baby* (1973)).

If the class has truly become a group and are now on easy terms with the teacher and each other, they may get the most benefit simply from being asked what they would like to talk about. If stimulating conversation dries up the leader might like to put any of the following questions.

'*What changes do you think the baby will bring in your life?*' This can lead to a useful discussion on arranging activities, preplanning to make housekeeping more simple, enlisting help from husbands, grandparents, friends. Suggestions can be made for preventing undue fatigue and the depression which often comes with it, and helping other children to accept the baby.

'*What sort of parents do you think you will be, disciplinarian or permissive?*' Do you think you can find a happy medium between allowing the baby to rule the household or being made to conform rigidly?

'*Do you think you will love your baby all the time?*' It is helpful to describe the mother's emotional see-saw between the baby's demands which are often expressed in apparently irrational crying, her drive to meet these needs as well as those of the rest of the family, and her occasional longing to be free to live her own life again. Mention can be made of the father's ambivalence between pride in his offspring and jealousy of his wife's involvement with it at the expense of his comfort and companionship, and of his feelings of responsibility towards his growing family with an occasional glance backwards to the carefree days of batchelorhood. Suggestions can be offered on handling interfering or possessive grandparents.

'*For what problems do you think you should seek help?*' When multigravidae are in the group, or members of a previous class have been invited to return to share their problems and solutions, many things will be mentioned which primigravidae, often dreaming of 'the perfect baby' will not have considered.

We must realise here that they also have ideals of being 'the perfect mother', and we can perhaps mention the late Dr D. W. Winnicott's comforting statement that a baby does not need perfection—that an 'ideal' mother would not prepare him for the world. He needs a 'good-enough' mother. When this is discussed, the group often decides that it will be all right to be a 'good enough' wife also. Many problems arise by trying too hard.

The biggest problem is usually crying. The cries of a baby are insistent, pathetic, urgent—and we don't know when he will stop. Music by the cot does help, and there are now cassettes of 'womb-music' which are often soothing. Recently, one of us has been visiting the mother of twins, and we both noticed that every time one baby was crying, she would stop to listen when the other made a noise. Other mothers tried the experiment of taping their own baby's murmuring sounds, together with their own voice talking softly, or singing. It has worked quite often—the tape is put on, and the baby stops crying, and listens. We mention this as it costs nothing, and even if it doesn't work all the time, it is worth trying.

Here, listed, are some problems which have been discussed in our own classes, most of them mentioned first by a member of the group, some by the teacher. The suggested sources of help are by no means arbitrary, but many parents find their own solutions, or seek help from family and close friends.

Problems of the mother
—painful breasts or perineum
—continuing postnatal 'blues'
—real depression
—constant tiredness
—not sleeping, even when she has the opportunity to rest
—disliking, or fearing to handle, her baby for more than 24 hours
—wishing to hurt the baby
—feeling 'always in a muddle', never getting a routine
—fearing her figure will never be back to normal, feeling unattractive.

Problems of the baby—*minor*
—breast hardness
—crying, being 'difficult to wind'
—'evening colic' or 'three-month colic'
—not sleeping in night
—constipation
—nappy rash
—'cradle-cap'
—not gaining weight
—gaining too much weight
—thrush
—'sticky eyes'
—infected umbilicus
—slight rashes of all kinds
—'taking ages to feed'.

Problems of the baby—*major*
—neonatal cold syndrome
—diarrhoea
—refusing feeds, especially when apathetic or with weak crying
—listess, fretful, persistent crying, even after feeds
—regular vomiting with failure to thrive
—signs of a painful ear, especially if discharging
—fever

—breathing difficulties, severe cold, cough, croup
—signs of abdominal pain, drawing up legs, continuous crying
—any accidents (home safety stressed here).

Problems of the family
—husband feeling neglected
—sexual difficulties; for example, painful intercourse, loss of libido
—housing difficulties
—financial worries.

Sources of help

General practitioner: major baby problems; problems of mother or
   family.
Health visitor: minor baby problems, referring when necessary;
   problems of mother or family.
Social workers: problems of mother or family (especially with
   housing and financial problems).
Voluntary organisations: see addresses in bibliography for
   specialities.
Hospital: any problems referred from the family doctor.
Physiotherapist: figure problems, muscle restoration, referred from
   general practitioner.
'*How do you think you will feel about making love again?*'   This
question is rarely raised spontaneously unless the group have
become very relaxed but there is usually an immediate response to
a discussion of the best time to resume intercourse, changes in
libido, the need for a gentle approach to overcome soreness of breasts
or from stitches. This can lead to a further question, 'At this
moment how many children do you think you would like to have
and at what intervals?' Answers from the group soon make it obvious
that each will need family planning advice. This is readily available
at family planning clinics, postnatal clinics and with family doctors,
though in some cases appointments take time to arrange. In some
hospitals mothers are interviewed during the lying-in period but this
is not a time when a woman is thinking very clearly and in any case
it must be a joint decision. A discussion initiated during pregnancy
gives the parents a preview of up-to-date methods and their use in
different circumstances. They can then think about the acceptability
and reliability of the different methods calmly before there is any
need for action.

Some teachers will begin this subject by showing a short film, such as 'Happy Family Planning', or a filmstrip (see appropriate section of this book for suggestions), at an evening parents' meeting. This can be followed by a further daytime class for the women alone, when all the products available can be demonstrated and handled, and non-mechanical methods mentioned for those with religious or other objections to appliances, spermicides or pills. Family planning clinics now make no charge. This makes it easier for a breast-feeding mother to be fitted at first with a diaphragm cap, or to obtain free supplies of sheaths and aerosol foams if she intends to take one of the contraceptive pills after she has weaned the baby.

This subject must be treated sensitively, giving clear descriptions, and being prepared to answer questions, while at the same time making it perfectly clear that the decision is the parents' own, in conjunction with their medical advisers.

In this class, as in most others, it is often appreciated if the teacher remains behind as the group disperses, so that individual problems can be discussed privately by any member wishing to do so.

REFERENCES

Creery, R. D. G. (1973) Infant nutrition and obesity. *Nursing Mirror*, **136**, (4) 34.
Darke, S. J. (1977) Changing trends in feeding the newborn baby. *Journal of the Institute of Health Education*, **15** (3), 6–10.
Klaus, *et al.* (1972) Child separation. *New England Journal of Medicine*, **286**, 460–463. Reprinted in *Pulse*, **24**, 25.
Montgomery, E. (1969) *At Your Best for Birth and Later*, p. 64. Bristol: Wright.
Report on Health and Social Subjects (1974) *Present Day Practice in Infants' Feeding*, No. 9. London: HMSO.
Whittlestone, W. H. (1977) The value of human milk. *Federation of New Zealand Parents Centre Bulletin*, Autumn 77, 5–9.
Winn, F. (1981) *New Baby*, p. 43. B. Edsall & Co under the authority of the Health Visitors' Association.
Winnicot D. W. (1966) *Maturational Processes and Facilitating Environments*. London: Tavistock Publications.
Tylden, E. (1975) Psychological and social considerations in breast feeding. *Journal of Human Nutrition*, **30**, 239–244.

FOR FURTHER READING

Infant feeding
Gunther, M. (1973) *Infant Feeding*. Harmondsworth: Penguin.
Hull, S. (1979) *Cooking for a Baby*. Harmondsworth: Penguin.
Scowen, P. & Wells, J. (1981) *Feeding Children in the First Year*. London: D. Edsall and Co.
Wood, C. & Smith, D. W. (1969) *MacKeith's Infant Feeding and Feeding Difficulties*, 6th edn. Edinburgh: Churchill Livingstone.

Breast feeding

Eiger, M. & Olds, S. W. (1973) *The Complete Book of Breast Feeding*. London: Bantam.

Helsing, E. & Savage King, F. (1982) *Breast Feeding in Practice*. Oxford: Oxford University Press.

Mackeith, R. (1969) Breast fed for the first two months. *Developmental Medicine and Child Neurology*, 11, 277–78.

Raphael, D. (1976) *The Tender Gift—Breastfeeding*. Schocken Books: New York.

Stables, J. (1981) *A Mother's Guide to Breastfeeding*. London: Star Publications.

Stanway, A. & Stanway, P. (1978) *Breast is Best*. London: Pan Books.

Stanway, A. & Stanway, P. (1982) *The Breast*. London: Granada.

National Childbirth Trust leaflets

A list of the latest leaflets will be sent on request.

Baby care

Bower, T. (1977) *The Perceptual World of the Child*. London: Fontana.

Cobb, J. (1980) *Babyshock. A Mother's First Five Years*. London: Pilot Productions Ltd.

Hardiment, C. (1983) *Dream Babies. A History of Childcare Manuals*. London: Jonathan Cape.

Hawkins, E. & Monro, K. (1977) *How to be a Supermum*. London: Van Dyke Books.

Illingworth, R. & Illingworth, C. (1977) *Babies and Young Children*, 6th edn. London: Churchill Livingstone.

Illingworth, R. S. (1983) *The Development of the Infant and Young Child—Abnormal and Normal*, 8th edn. Edinburgh: Churchill Livingstone.

Jolly, H. (1981) *Book of Child Care*, 3rd edn. London: George Allen and Unwin.

Jolly, H. (1978) *More Common Sense about Babies and Children*. London: Pelham Books.

Klaus, M. & Kennell, J. (1976) *Maternal-Infant Bonding*. London: Mosby. Obtainable ICEA.

Leach, P. (1974) *Babyhood*. London: Pelican.

Leach, P. (1977) *Baby and Child*. London: Michael Joseph.

MacLaughlin, C. J. *et al.* (1976) *The Black Parents' Handbook*. New York: Harcourt, Brace, Jovanovich.

Rayner, C. (1977) *Family Feelings (Understanding Your Child From 0–5)*. London Arrow Books in association with Health Education Council.

Schaffer, R. (1977) *Mothering*. London: Fontana.

Shapiro, J. (1977) *Good Housekeeping Baby Book*. London: Ebury Press.

Spock, B. (1971) *Baby and Child Care*. London: New English Library.

Stern, D. (1977) *The First Relationship—Infant and Mother*. London: Fontana.

Tucker, N. (1977) *What is a Child?* London: Fontana.

Winnicott, D. W. (1962) *The Child and the Family*. London: Tavistock.

Postnatal exercises

McLaren, J. (1980) *Preparing for Parenthood*. London: Murray.

McKenna, J., Polden, M. & Williams, M. (1980) *You After Childbirth*. Edinburgh: Churchill Livingstone.

Montgomery, E. (1969) *At Your Best for Birth and Later*. Bristol: Wright.

Noble, E.(1980) *Essential Exercises for the Childbearing Year* (English edition). London: Murray.

Miscellaneous

Andry, C. & Schepp, S. (1969) *How Babies are Made*. Time Life International.

Obtainable from Marriage Guidance Council, 76A New Cavendish Street, London W.1. Beautifully illustrated book for young children.

Barnes, J. (1976) *Essentials of Family Planning*. Oxford: Blackwell Scientific Publications.

Dalton, K. (1980) *Depression after Childbirth*. Oxford: Oxford University Press.

Montague, A. (1971) *Touching*. London: Harper & Row.

Booklets for parents (free from clinics and hospitals)

A New Beginning. L. R. Industries Ltd, North Circular Road, Chingford, London E4. A family planning booklet for Indian couples.

A Simple Guide to Bottle Feeding. Health Education Council.

Immunisation. Health Education Council.

Morris, N. F. (1972) *The Baby Book*, National Clinic edition. Newbourne Publications Ltd, Recorder House, Church Street, London N16.

Rayner, C. (1973) *Now You're a Family*. Health Education Council, 78 New Oxford Street, London WC1.

Rayner C. *You Know More Than You Think You Do*. Health Education Council.

SMA Breast and Bottle feeding Charts. Wyeth Parentcraft, Wyeth Laboratories, Huntercombe Lane South, Taplow, Maidenhead.

The Baby Blues and Post-Natal Depression. Health Education Council.

Winn, F. (1981) *First Three Years*. Health Visitors' Association, 36 Eccleston Square, London SW1.

Weston, T (1972) *You and Your Baby, Parts I and II*. Family Doctor Publications, 47–51 Chalton Street, London NW1.

Family doctor booklets (obtainable from 47–51 Chalton, Street, London NW1, for a small charge)

De Kok, W. (1961) *Understanding Your Child*.

Diack, H. (1965) *Learning to Talk and Read*.

Morris, W. I. C. (1965) *Letters to an Expectant Mother*.

Pilkington, R. (1972) *How Life Began*.

10

Fathers' evenings and film shows

In some parts of the world where marriages are arranged by parents, teenage boys and girls receive earnest instruction about how to conduct themselves as husbands, wives and citizens and the obligations they will later owe as parents to their families as well as to the tribe or nation. In western civilisation there is little preparation for marriage other than the criterion of romantic love and even less in the joys and responsibilities of parenthood. Important efforts are being made to overcome these defects in homes, schools and clubs but it will be a very long time before fathercraft competes with more academic subjects in the syllabuses of boys' schools. It is therefore hardly surprising that many men are abysmally ignorant about the facts of reproduction, not to mention their emotional overtones. Some men retreat from involvement in their wife's pregnancy, labour and care of their baby through fear of showing this ignorance; others are keen to overcome it and come willingly for interviews or classes.

There is no doubt that pregnancy may give rise to stress and anxiety in men as well as women. If the pregnancy was unplanned the man may feel trapped by his future responsibilities, particularly financial ones, and resentful about the coming curtailment of his freedom. Even if the baby is wanted, many men swing between joy in this fulfilment of their virility, anxiety about their wives and worry about their capabilities as fathers. A first pregnancy is particularly critical since it will certainly bring changes to the marriage relationship, the couple will no longer face the world as a pair, but will have to learn to live for many years in the close and demanding presence of another human being. In many cases this binds the marriage together and it develops a deeper and more meaningful relationship with the birth of each child, but occasionally a man, particularly one who sees his wife as a substitute mother, is jealous of his child. This puts a great strain on the marriage and in a few,

207

happily rare, instances the birth of a child is the final straw that breaks an unstable marriage.

Women are inundated with information and advice about pregnancy but men will find very little in books or magazines written expressly to help them. The number of full preparation classes open to couples is small, there are some single classes available during early pregnancy and a fathers' class during late pregnancy is now fairly common. Many men now take advantage of these classes, but many more will not do so through selfconsciousness or fear of being regarded as unmanly, their sole means of learning being therefore through their mates at work, their female relations, or second-hand through their wife's classes.

It is inevitable that a man experiences his wife's pregnancy at second hand. The changes in her body gradually help a woman to accept pregnancy and come to know something of her baby. With the exception of the baby's movements which may delight him when they are lying together, the man can only observe and not feel. It takes a loving and sympathetic husband to enter into all the hopes and fears of his pregnant wife and to accept her mood swings, changes in libido and changes in shape. Some husbands treat their wives as if they are made of Dresden china and become over-protective or even dictatorial, while others try to pretend the pregnancy does not exist and expect their wives to behave accordingly.

The father's role in labour has changed through the ages in different countries and is in a state of flux in our own society today. The 'couvade syndrome' in which the man took to his bed with simulated labour pains and received a great deal of care and attention while his wife went off quietly by herself to give birth to her baby was common in ancient Greece and parts of Africa. In other countries it was the custom for the husband to help his wife in labour, for example in Malaya the peasants sit cross-legged behind their wives to support them in the second stage. In Victorian and Edwardian England the whole process of childbearing and rearing, except for the disciplining of unruly offspring, was considered to be the woman's responsibility. It was only after the first world war, and more rapidly since 1945, that men's and women's roles in our society have been changing and growing closer together. Today young people share every aspect of their lives, they work together, play together, housekeep together, it is hardly surprising that many of them wish to be together when the child they have jointly conceived is born. Some couples are temperamentally unsuited to such a situation and it certainly raises problems for hospital staff, but once they have become used to the idea most observers say that they believe that both men and women derive great benefit from it. In a study done at Charing Cross Hospital, Pawson and Morris (1971) found that 92% of 730 husbands felt that their presence in labour was beneficial to their wives. Raising of morale, improving physical comfort, assistance in carrying out training and improvement of the husband-wife relationship were the reasons offered by the men.

More recently a prospective study of 45 couples was undertaken by Drähne et al (1977) in Tubingen. 'The couples were given detailed questionnaires 4–6 weeks before delivery, they were systematically observed for the last two hours before delivery, and on the 5th to 6th day afterwards were interviewed separately.' 'A very close statistical relationship was shown between the success of the man and of his wife. The preparation beforehand played a very important role at the successful outcome at delivery.'

When asked how they felt in the labour room half the men replied that during the first stage they were unsure of themselves and noticed signs of tension. Some were bored and felt useless and helpless. The authors note the importance of these answers and state that special preparations before the birth can prevent these manifestations, though they do not tell us how they do this. During the actual delivery three-quarters of the men said they felt better because they, as well as their wives, could be more active.

When asked 'Do you believe the relationship to your partner has changed due to this experience?' almost every man replied 'Yes'. Feelings of admiration and thankfulness were very prevalent. Furthermore the majority of the men believed they would develop a more positive relationship to the child and 'accept the new role as a father more easily.'

If a man is to give real support to his wife rather than be just a sympathetic and possibly worried onlooker, he must understand something about the process and management of labour and how she may react to them. It is for this reason that some hospitals insist that fathers should attend one or two preparation classes if they wish to be present at the birth of their child. We strongly believe that these classes, if held early enough, can also help men to become more involved in planning for their baby and in making pregnancy a happier time for each of the couple. Many women have said to us after a fathers' class that their husbands were much more interested in their progress and ready to discuss it. Having discovered that labour is not all blood and pain and that there is a great deal they can do to help, they had changed their minds about attending it.

Classes on baby care and child rearing are still only available to a very small minority of men. It is to be hoped that more groups such as those described by Aline Auerbach (1967) in her book *Parents Learn Through Group Discussion* in cooperation with the Child Study Association of America, will be started in this country. Perhaps, then, more men and women will come to realise how their own behaviour influences the physical and mental development of their children and lays the foundation for their future family life.

FATHERS' CLASSES

Planning of these evenings will be determined by the numbers to be catered for and the facilities available. We have chosen to describe two types: first, two classes which are part of a course for a small group of eight to 12 mothers and, secondly, a film evening open to a large group of parents, some of whom may be attending other classes. Careful organisation is needed for any of these meetings: date and time must be advertised well beforehand so that husbands can arrange to be free on that night, clear instructions must be given on how to get to the venue which may well be different from the antenatal clinic premises; and on the evening clear signposts to the hall and the nearest lavatories are important. Mothers often ask beforehand for an outline of the class including a description of any slides or films which may be shown, and the teacher or any member of the antenatal team should be ready to give this information and mention that if any husband dislikes a picture that is shown nobody will think any the worse of him if he steps out for a smoke. If partners cannot attend, then mothers, sisters or friends should be welcome. Some estimate of the likely numbers is needed so that sufficient chairs can be provided without the room being uncomfortably crowded.

Several assistants are needed for a large group, and even for a small one at least one helper is useful to talk to parents, project slides or make coffee. A couple who have recently had a baby, particularly if the man has been at the labour, make ideal helpers. The room must be prepared well in advance: a large group requires formal rows but for a small group it looks more friendly if the lines of chairs are curved or, if slides are not being used, are arranged in a circle. Good ventilation is particularly important since pregnant women are sensitive to a crowded stuffy atmosphere and both they and their husbands may be somewhat apprehensive, especially if a birth film is being shown. Having run through the film to check for breaks or having focused a slide projector it is often a good idea in summer to open windows and leave the room unblacked until the last moment.

We believe that couples should be met at the door by the teacher or her helpers and made to feel welcome rather than being left to drift into an unfamiliar room; they should also be encouraged to fill up blocks of seats leaving some empty ones near the door for the latecomers. A selection of leaflets scattered on the chairs gives the early arrivals something to do and, while exchanging them, the ice is often broken; it must, however, be made clear whether the leaflets are free or must be paid for if people wish to take them away at the end of the evening. In the latter case, a box and a plentiful supply of small change must be available. Refreshments in the form of coffee, tea, or cold drinks and biscuits are a tremendous help in making the evening more sociable, but the cost for a large group is quite high and may need to be subsidised by the Health Service or the parents. If these are being served, careful preparation is again the watchword but husbands will be only too ready to hand round and help clear up. A chair and a glass of water conveniently placed outside the hall is a wise precaution on film evenings, and young helpers, perhaps student midwives, to be with the fathers and reassure them.

A plan for the first class for a small group

Introductions—it may be interesting to include jobs, since two men may well find that they have this bond in common, but this may be undesirable if the group is intellectually very mixed

The teacher may wish to add a few words about the clinic, hospital or society such as the National Childbirth Trust which is responsible for the meeting.

A short talk on the physical and emotional changes of pregnancy illustrated with charts, pelvis, doll or slides or a filmstrip such as 'Your First Baby, Part 1', 'The Expectant Father,' or 'Pregnancy— a Challenging Experience'. Questions and comments welcomed throughout as well as at the end.

Coffee break.

Points about antenatal care if not already covered by filmstrip or film, leading to a discussion on how the group view pregnancy and their daily activities. Minor aches and pains, emotional ups and downs.

The value of preparation classes, with a review of what else they will cover. If the women are already booked into a course this can be very brief, just enough to arouse the men's interest in what their wives will be learning but, if not, a fuller description is needed for propaganda purposes.

A demonstration of good posture, lifting, etc., and some contraction and relaxation exercises while sitting on chairs can illustrate some of these points and cause amusement and a lighthearted atmosphere.

A brief discussion on plans for the baby. Baby clothes are boring to men but their interest can usually be aroused in prams, cots, the height of working surfaces and where the baby is going to sleep.

Finally, the teacher should note the names of any women who are not already booked into subsequent classes and announce the dates and times of further classes including the second evening for fathers, visits to the wards or talks by additional speakers. She should thank the members of the group for coming and bid them goodnight. If she has succeeded in making a good rapport with the group she will get offers of help with the clearing up and should allow at least 15 minutes extra time for the one or two couples who are likely to want a word in private.

Second class for fathers towards the end of the course

If the group have already met they will be happy to renew acquaintanceship and exchange notes, otherwise introductions will be needed.

Talk on the physiology and management of labour illustrated with blackboard, charts, knitted uterus, baby and box or pelvis, slides or filmstrip such as 'Your First Baby, Part 2' or 'Birth, a Shared Experience'. If colour slides of an actual delivery are used points about the mother's expression in the second stage, blood-stained liquor, the appearance of the baby and anything else the teacher has discovered that worries parents (these she will only discover from experience) should be described *before* the picture is projected. Questions and comments welcomed throughout.

Further questions and comments initiated by the teacher on the lines of: What did you think of those pictures? Were any points not clear? Did anything worry you?

It is not a bad idea to leave out some important piece of information from the talk, for example when to call the midwife or go into hospital, as this is a question uppermost in most men's minds and may well give rise to a first question.

Coffee break.

Practical hints on husband's help. This can be done as a talk—see suggestions at the end of the chapter—but is much more vivid and useful if done in the form of a brief labour rehearsal. The husbands check the different kinds of relaxation and breathing, learn back and tummy massage and various forms of support. If the teacher feels that she or the parents will be embarrassed by this it is possible to rehearse timed contractions sitting on chairs with the husbands checking their wives. The teacher and her helper can demonstrate massage for the first stage and breathing for the second stage but a demonstration is never so effective as actually trying out the skill.

Discussion usually flows freely but is greatly helped if there is at least one husband present who has had experience of his wife in labour.

Finally, a brief discussion on 'afterwards'. If slides have not been used during the first part of the evening, 'Your First Baby, Part 3' or the film 'With a Little Help' and, in the presence of multigravidae, 'More Tiny Feet' may make a useful starting point. Failing these, a question to an experienced father or a general enquiry as to 'what do you think life will be like after the birth?' will usually get things going. This can lead to a few words about excitements, discomforts and mood swings in the puerperium in hospital and later at home. The wife's need for help in the first few weeks with domestic chores while she learns to cope with the baby, the husband's role in supporting and encouraging her, and the introduction of the baby to grandparents and other children, are all topics to be covered. Then there should be a look into the future when a reliable baby sitter must be found, and the wife detached from the baby for a few hours so that the couple can begin to go out together again.

The evening can end with good wishes and reminders of ways the group can keep in touch with the teacher and each other, such as letters, phone calls, visits or whatever may be appropriate to the group. Some groups will know, for instance, that they will be having a postnatal reunion. This is usually enjoyed very much and may lead to more lasting friendships.

COUPLES' CLASSES

Some husbands come to fathers' evenings rather unwillingly only after considerable pressure from their wives, but they book up for a couples' class only if they have a close relationship with their partner and are already deeply involved in her pregnancy; they make a highly receptive audience. The class syllabus is not likely to vary greatly from those already discussed though a thorough knowledge of the male as well as the female reproductive system is essential. However the fact that one has more time with the men makes the teacher's approach somewhat different. During a course including one or even two fathers' evenings the time is largely taken up with trying to help the men understand their partners' reactions, now they can be encouraged to explore their own. For example, one can try such questions as 'How do you feel about becoming a father?' 'How do you enjoy your baby's movements?' 'How do *you* react to pain or stress?' 'How do you think you will feel about making love again?' or 'How much do you plan to share the baby's care?'. These can stimulate very lively discussion.

During the practical sessions the couple work together as a team, they all learn the breathing, relaxation and massage techniques so that they can both appreciate the required sensations and skills. Attendance at such classes is usually very good but if one husband has some other commitment the teacher can usually play his part or another man will offer to help two women for that evening. It is particularly important that there should be a break in such a class when the teacher is doing something else and the couples can talk informally among themselves. They will get to know each other, perhaps plan to go out for a drink or a meal and it is not unusual for lifelong friendships to be started in this way.

It is very helpful to introduce to the group a new father who is prepared to discuss with them his reaction to his wife's labour and his feelings immediately after the birth, when perhaps he had to go home to an empty house. He will often be prepared to talk about the changes in his life and his response to sharing his wife with his baby

It is very encouraging that recently, evening courses for couples are being offered in many hospitals.

FILM EVENINGS

Ideally, parents should come to classes and look at black-and-white pictures and see colour slides of a birth before they make up their minds that they wish to see a film, but unfortunately this is not always possible. Colour films of birth, no matter what angle they are filmed from, are emotional dynamite; they may be reassuring but, on the other hand, they can do a great deal of harm. It is not always easy for doctors and midwives, to whom birth is a common experience, to appreciate its impact on a lay audience. Professionals naturally look first for good midwifery technique, while the audience look first at the expressions on the parents' faces and the appearance of the baby. Some of the parents may have seen birth films at school or on television but that is a very different matter from picturing themselves in a few weeks' time playing the roles of the man or woman on the screen. A few notes on films currently available in this country will be found in the Appendix, although the ideal film has not yet been made and perhaps never will be.

Films are expensive to hire and require skilled projection, and there may therefore be a temptation to try out a new film on an audience. We make no apologies for saying that no teacher should show a film to an audience of parents unless she has seen it several times herself and is in broad agreement with its sentiments; she can then introduce the film in an interesting way, perhaps saying a little about its history, giving reasons for a particular procedure or suggesting some special point to look out for. It is possible to lower the emotional temperature of the meeting in this way. For example, in the film 'The Waiting Game' the audience should perhaps be warned that after a rather sentimental beginning, in which husbands and wives examine their feelings towards the end of pregnancy, the film ends with four deliveries each one accompanied by a great deal of hard work and what appears to be a lot of pain for the mother. The husband is shown making a great emotional contribution and sharing in the delight, overwhelming relief and extreme joy afterwards. Husbands should be advised that their presence with their wives at this turning point in their lives is very important, but that every human being shows emotion differently and that their wives will know this.

When a film is finished there need be no hurry to turn the lights on and it is often a good idea to suggest that parents discuss it among themselves while the film is rewound. Then the teacher can ask if there are any questions and wait quietly for a few minutes while the first one is formulated.

A film evening for a large audience

One of us (D.B.) is concerned with a film evening for up to 100 parents held in the lecture theatre of a hospital medical centre, where informality and personal contact is achieved by breaking up the large audience into small groups for tea or coffee and discussion. For this film evening the expectant parents are from several local classes, and from the hospital's own classes. It is held regularly so that the couples attending have a choice of dates. However, it is preferred that they attend towards the end of the wife's class sessions, when we hope they will have practised techniques together and become familiar with the pattern of labour. The dates are given to the women well ahead, so that their husbands can arrange to be free, but it is emphasised that if the thought of a film is really off-putting to either of them, they should not attend.

Clear directions are given on the location of the Medical Centre within the hospital complex. When the couple arrive at the door, they are greeted by student midwives, who show them to the lecture theatre, where other staff and local antenatal teachers are waiting to ensure that everybody is comfortably seated. Five minutes are allowed for latecomers, and when everybody has settled in, one of the senior hospital sisters gives a short talk.

First, she welcomes everybody to the hospital and reassures husbands that they are accepted warmly by the hospital staff when their wives are in labour. However, she makes the point that if their wives are in very early labour when admitted, and especially if they are to be sedated for the night, husbands may be asked to go home for a while. They can, if they wish, then phone in often, or will be telephoned by the hospital when their wives need them.

A brief reminder is given about when to come to hospital and of the routine of ringing the hospital first, before getting the ambulance, so that staff are prepared for the wife's admission. Husbands are warned that they will have to wear a white gown and a mask and told that, if they wish, they can sit on a stool by their wife's left shoulder as the baby is born, thus seeing very little more of the birth than their wife will see. If they wish to see the baby's head as it first appears, they can go to the bottom of the bed and do so. Alternatively, as wives need support especially at the end of the first stage, and several members of staff will be with her in the second stage to help, he need not feel guilty if he 'sits out' for this part and returns immediately the baby is born.

She ends by asking for the husbands' help after the film to move tables which are stacked at the back of the room, and arrange chairs round them, so that informal groups of couples can be formed in different parts of the room. She says that a member of the staff or a local antenatal teacher will be at each table to answer any questions or discuss interesting points in the film, and that tea, coffee or fruit drinks, with biscuits, will be served at the tables (a small charge is made for this).

One of the antenatal teachers then introduces a film briefly. (See film list). The point is always made that a film watched is often more traumatic than a delivery witnessed, because in the delivery the husband becomes part of the helping team, has an active role, and is excited at the imminent birth of his baby. As the birth is usually filmed from the foot of the bed, husbands are told this, and reminded again that they need not see this angle in real life at all unless they wish to do so. Husbands are also encouraged to take their jackets off and make themselves comfortable (the room is always very warm and it would be a pity if they felt slightly squeamish simply because of the heat). The point is emphasised again that any questions, however small or seemingly trivial, will be answered later.

After the film all the staff help the husbands sort out the tables and chairs. This seems to be a good tension-relieving activity and adds to the casual attitude and friendliness of the small groups. The student midwives serve the drinks, then join the groups and often help in answering queries.

The sister or antenatal teacher at each table usually begins by eliciting comments on the film and asks how many of the husbands wish to be with their wives in labour, and if the film has influenced or changed the decision in any way. We discuss the ways in which a husband can help his wife throughout labour, and by this time the group usually provides its own impetus and discussion flows easily.

Husbands almost always ask for a repetition of the different signs that their wives are ready for hospital. Occasionally we are asked what they should do with a precipitate delivery at home. Usually they say they had not realised how much help they could give, and are determined to practise more with their wives at home.

If the question is not asked in any form, each group is told very clearly about postnatal 'blues' and approximately when they occur. Special emphasis is also made of the fact that any woman will be very tired on return from hospital, and will need a period of time in which all household chores are taken care of, so that she can devote herself to getting used to the baby, planning a routine, and resting to make up for disturbed nights. Each couple is asked what arrangements they have made for this and, if none, whether there is a possibility of husband, sister, mother or mother-in-law 'taking over' the daily routine of the house for a period of one to two weeks. Husbands are told that, by allowing their wives this time for recovery, weariness will pass quickly, but if she has to cope alone from the beginning she may be very tired for months.

The length of discussion varies from half an hour to over an hour, depending on the wishes of the group. As each disperse, at different times, the staff make them feel they have been glad to see them, and will be welcoming when they arrive for delivery.

SOME OF THE THINGS A FATHER CAN DO TO HELP

Here is an outline of a brief talk to fathers which could follow a description of labour.

'You may both find the last few weeks of pregnancy a bit trying, your wife getting heavy and tired and both of you on edge, half longing for the day when all the waiting will be over, half dreading the beginning of labour. Do plan some short excursions, maybe a meal out, the last time for a long time that you can do these things without a baby-sitter, and encourage visitors providing they don't cause too much work. There is nothing worse for the morale than sitting around all day with nothing to do, feeling like an "unexploded bomb", although it is important to get enough rest.

'Encourage your wife to go on practising each day any exercises that she has learned and help by talking her through a pretend contraction (see Ch. 6) and checking her breathing and relaxation. One doesn't have to be too serious about it all, you are not trying to pass an examination in "How to have a baby", but don't destroy her confidence by teasing.

'After tonight I hope you will both be quite clear about when to go into hospital or to call the midwife. Check that you have a list of the required telephone numbers, 10p pieces for a telephone, petrol, oil, water and a couple of cushions in the car if you are bringing her in yourself. If you are planning to stay you may be glad of some emergency rations, for although hospitals are good about cups of tea, the odd apple or biscuit can help a lot during a long waiting period. If you are still feeling doubtful about your staying powers do remember that nobody is going to turn a key on you. Unlike your wife you are free to come and go, and in any case the hospital authorities will reserve the right to ask you to leave the room on certain occasions.

'When labour starts let your wife enjoy the natural excitement but calm her down if she is dashing around too much. If you go into hospital together you will be asked to sit in a waiting room while your wife is examined in the admission ward; if labour is progressing she may be "prepared" with an examination and bath. She will then go to a ward or first-stage room where you can join her. By now her contractions may be a good deal stronger and require real concentration on her part. If they are becoming painful she will tend to fight them by tensing her body, screwing up her face and holding her breath. Her first line of defence is to relax and go with the contraction, doing the breathing that she has been taught and allowing her uterus to get on with its job. You can help enormously, first of all simply by being a familiar presence among strange surroundings, secondly by helping her to concentrate and keep going. The midwives will be very kind and will come in and out but they may have several women in labour to look after, while you will only have one. You can arrange supports and pillows to keep your wife comfortable, give her frequent sips of fluid if this is allowed, massage her back or tummy and sponge her face and hands with cold water. At first your wife will probably be glad to talk in between contractions or ask you to read to her if she cannot be bothered with a book herself, but later she will wish to stay quiet. Rest a hand on hers during contractions, for if she is holding yours she will tend to grip it and squeeze you instead of relaxing. Remember you are there to help your wife. Don't give all your attention to the monitoring machines!

'If she is given pills or an injection and seems to be truly asleep, have a snooze yourself if it is at night and let her be. If she wakes at the height of each contraction and seems to panic, time them carefully, and when you know she is about due for another watch for the tense hands or screwed-up face which are early signs of discomfort, then wake her gently and encourage her to get into her breathing rhythm before the contraction takes hold of her. In any case, the midwives will be glad to have your record of the time intervals between contractions. At some stage she is likely to say that she just cannot go on and this is when she will need all *your* strength, *your* trust in the staff and belief in what she has learned. Breathe with her, tap with her, count for her, hand her the gas and oxygen if she is using it. Don't be hurt if she suddenly gets bad-tempered, maybe changes from telling you how wonderful you are to grumbling that it is all your fault. This is the time to watch for signs of the end of the first stage, strong frequent contractions, a feeling of fullness in the bowel and the beginning of the pushing urge. If you are alone together and you notice she is catching her breath or grunting at the height of a contraction, see her through that one by encouraging her to blow out into the mask or to do the broken rhythm breathing (blow, in, blow) then go and find a midwife and report what is happening.

'While the midwife is examining her, slip along to the lavatory, then have a good wash so that you'll be ready to go into the labour ward if you wish. Remember that labour wards tend to be hot and you will be excited, so strip down to a thin cotton shirt before putting on the gown, cap and mask that you will be offered.

'Once she is settled in the delivery room there will be a number of people around helping your wife, but remember she may still need *your* presence and the added encouragement of *your* voice. You may also be able to help by holding the pillows, which tend to slip, or lifting her with an arm round her shoulders when she is pushing or supporting one leg while a midwife holds the other. At a home delivery where the midwife may be single-handed these efforts are particularly appreciated.

'If you can spare a minute from the top end you'll be able to catch a glimpse of your baby's head as it comes down and round the birth canal and cheer your wife on by reporting on how much you can see. Listen very carefully to the midwife or doctor, so that at the critical moment when the head is being born and they say, "Don't push any more, open your mouth and pant", you can reiterate straight into your wife's ear, "Let go, darling, and pant".

'There can be few more exciting moments in a man's life than to be the first to tell his wife the sex of their child.'

REFERENCES

Auerbach, A. (1967) *Parents Learn Through Group Discussion*. New York: Wiley.
Drahne A., Doch S., König S. & Zubke W. (1977) *The Husband's Presence at Delivery a Prospective Study*. In 5th International Congress of Psychosomatic Obstetrics & Gynecology, 20B pp 897–899. London: Academic Press.
Pawson, M. & Morris, N. (1971) The role of the father in pregnancy and labour. *Third International Congress of Psychosomatic Medicine in Obstetrics and Gynaecology*, p. 273. Basel: Karger.

FOR FURTHER READING

Bing, E. & Colman, L. (1978) *Making Love during Pregnancy*. London: Bantam Books.
Bradley, R. (1965) *Husband-Coached Childbirth*. London: Harper & Row. Obtainable ICEA.
Karitane Mothercraft Society (1977) *An Approach to Fatherhood*. Sydney: Randwick.
Kitzinger, S. (1973) *Giving Birth—The Parents' Emotions in Childbirth*. London: Sphere Books.
Little, P. & Ralston, D. (1980) *The Baby Book for Dads*. London: New English Library.
Maternity Center Association, *For the Expectant Father*. 48 East 92nd Street, New York 10028.
Mayle, P. (1980) *How to be a Pregnant Father*. London: Macmillan.
Mckee, L. & O'Brien, M. (ed.) (1982) *The Father Figure*. London: Tavistock.
National Childbirth Trust (1976) *Expectant Father's Leaflet*, No. 9.
Parke, R. D. (1981) *Fathering*. London: Fontana.

Parsons, B. (1982) *The Expectant Father*. Quatermaine House, Windmill Road, Sunbury on Thames, Middlesex.

Schaeffer, G. (1972) *The expectant Father*. London: Harper & Row. Obtainable ICEA.

Free leaflet

It's Your Baby Too. Wyeth Laboratories, Taplow, Maidenhead, Berks.

11

The value of antenatal education

In Chapter 1 it was stated that the aims of antenatal education were as follows:

1. To give a woman more confidence.
2. To help her to have a healthy, happy pregnancy and a speedy rehabilitation afterwards.
3. To prepare her for the reality of labour.
4. To integrate her into a group having similar problems to her own
5. To begin to prepare her to care for her baby.

It is very difficult to assess the effects of any form of health education, particularly one largely concerned with mental well-being, but in this chapter we shall look at some of the evidence that we have as to whether or not these aims are being achieved. Most of the work that has been done concerns the effect of training on labour, and the results are very contradictory, but some studies have been undertaken into other aspects of classes. The evidence submitted here is drawn from various papers referred to at the end of the chapter and from a large scale review of 'Preparation for Parenthood' sponsored by the Royal College of Midwives in 1966. The second part of this study was conducted by a national field survey of representative samples of 1230 mothers of first babies, 284 expectant mothers and a series of group discussions under the guidance of a psychologist. The full report should be read by all concerned with the care of expectant parents, as there is only space here to select a few figures.

In this country where attendance at classes is often not actively encouraged and patients are self-selected, there is a general consensus of opinion that it is the more anxious women who go to classes, but Mandelstam (1971) found that those who attended the classes in her survey did not have a higher introversion rating on the Eysenck personality scale than non-attenders.

Results of attempts to build up confidence

In the Royal College of Midwives' Survey (1966, p. 44) approximately 95% of mothers in the antenatal sample found the classes generally helpful. The courses were somewhat arbitrarily divided into three groups: relaxation and exercise classes made up Group A, pregnancy and labour classes Group B, and baby care Group C. To the specific question 'Did the classes give confidence generally?' the answer was 'yes' for 63% of women attending Group A classes, 66% for those attending Group B classes, and 4% in Group C. Similar results were found by Rathbone (1970) who said that when mothers were asked 'How did you find the classes?' they often stressed the extra confidence which the preparation gave them. She found that women trained by some teachers found labour worse than expected while other groups trained by different teachers found it better. She points out that this is probably a reflection of the different tenor of the teaching, some of which was realistic, some perhaps oversanguine. These findings were challenged by Mandelstam (1971) who found that 'attendance at classes did not appear to make any serious difference to the state of mind of the patient on admission'.

Health and happiness during pregnancy

There is very little valid evidence about the effect of classes on pregnancy. Chertok (1959) quotes comparative statistics from various authors on the occurrence of toxaemia, including one from Choupik, the Minister of Health of the Soviet Union. This report, from 10 hospitals in the Moscow region, gives the number of women having late toxaemias as 3.65% among those receiving psychoprophylaxis compared with 6.8% in others.

There is now good evidence that at least one problem during pregnancy, namely backache, can be helped by antenatal education and exercises. In 1977, Mantle *et al* found that 48% of a sample of 180 women delivered at the London hospital had backache during pregnancy; in one third of these it was severe. In 1981, the same team found that a group of 85 women given back care advice similar to that used in 'back pain schools' early in pregnancy had a significantly lower amount of backache than those in a control group.

We have no statistical evidence that pre- and postnatal exercises improve the condition of the pelvic floor and prevent complications due to weakness, though clinical observation suggests that they do.

We now have some evidence that frequent pelvic floor contractions diminish the incidence of stress incontinence in older women. S. Harrison writing in a *Textbook of Physiotherapy in some Surgical Conditions* (Cash, 1979) describes a group of 212 patients with stress incontinence as their main symptom, 16 of whom had already had failed repairs. These patients were taught a strict routine of pelvic floor exercises; 199 had no further incontinence, while only 13 failed to respond.

Happiness during pregnancy, or at any other time, is impossible to measure, but the RCM survey (1966, p. 34) showed that 84% of the women in the antenatal sample were unhappy about some aspect of their pregnancies. The greatest fear, held by 54%, was of having an abnormal baby, 35% were frightened of 'the unknown generally', 29% were frightened of 'making a fool of myself', and 25% of pain. When asked what had helped them most with their worries, 32% said classes, 22% said reassurance from family and friends, and only 15% said professional reassurance (p. 35).

Effects on labour

In 1965, at a meeting at St Anne's College, Oxford, Professor Peter Huntingford was asked to sum up from the published literature the objective results of training on labour (Conference Report of Obstetric Association of Chartered Physiotherapists, p. 21). He felt that a number of different methods of preparation were concerned and the details were not always adequately described. Several reliable studies of the effects on the complications of labour had been described, but objective observations of the length of labour, the amount of analgesia, and the assessment of pain had not been well controlled. He went on to discuss some of the reasons for these difficulties. The selection and matching of controls present great difficulty, as patients who choose to come to classes are usually self-selected. Non-attenders cannot be given a placebo, and presence of an observer, particularly one who has been concerned with any part of the training, is likely to influence the mother's behaviour. Measurement of the length of labour is another stumbling block, the normal range is very wide and the criteria for the onset of labour vary; trained women, if less anxious, may tend to present later. The amount of analgesics used is not neccessarily an indication of the pain felt. It is determined by several interacting factors; the mother's demands will vary according to her pain threshold, her personality, what she has heard about analgesics from her friends and in class, and the criteria for administration of analgesics in the unit. Professor Huntingford felt that an objective assessment of pain was possible only if based on very careful recording of contractions and the mother's reaction to them all through the active phase of labour.

Objective results. In spite of these difficulties a number of surveys have been done in this country and many more abroad, and they have had a marked effect on the training and handling of women in labour. Unfortunately, Grantly Dick-Read did not publish any surveys, but in 1954 Heardman, using preparation based on his methods, published the results of observations on 1000 primiparae, of whom 500 were trained and 500 untrained. They were matched for age and delivered in the same labour wards. It is noted that a physiotherapist was present at the birth of a large majority of the babies though it is not clear whether this applied to untrained as well as trained mothers. The average length of labour was 17 hours for the trained, 20 hours for the controls; the number of forceps deliveries was 47 from the trained, 86 for controls and the number of perineal tears and episiotomies was reduced from 3122 to 227 in the trained women.

These results have never been duplicated in this country and surveys by Roberts *et al.* (1953), Peel (1955), Burnett (1956) and latterly Mandelstam (1971) all show no significant difference between the prepared and unprepared groups, with the exception that Roberts found a difference in favour of the trained group in the amount of sedation required. Details of the training in these papers are scanty. Roberts described it as the 'Heardman' method, which included one introductory talk by a doctor. Peel and Burnett simply described the training as 'antenatal exercises'; how these exercises were used or how women were supported in labour was not discussed.

Subjective results. A few attempts have been made to evaluate the subjective results of preparation for labour, notably by Matthews (1965). He compared two matched groups of prepared and unprepared mothers though his criteria for 'preparation' was that the mothers in this group had 'attended at least one relaxation class'. The conditions for the administration of analgesia were carefully laid down and the amount used by each group was almost identical, but Matthews found that the prepared patients stood 'a better chance of a labour free from fear, were more likely to be cooperative, and only 4% of them, as against 23% of the unprepared mothers, found labour more painful than expected'. He concluded with the remark that 'it would probably be fair to say that these figures lend support to the suggestion that relaxation exercises are beneficial in relieving subjective symptoms'. He added that 'neither the writer nor the hospital staff have shown any positive enthusiasm for preparation and the unit itself could hardly be considered ideal for these methods; yet despite these negative approaches, the results appeared to be significant! One wonders how much more significant they would be if physiotherapist, midwife and doctor took more interest in each other's work; attempting, perhaps, to standardise instructions to women in labour.'

These surveys, from such centres as King's College Hospital, Hammersmith Hospital and the West Middlesex Hospital, have had a profound effect on obstetric thinking in this country during the last 20 years; they are in great contrast to the reports of psychoprophylactic preparation on the continent and in South America.

Results from abroad. Chertok (1959) gave a large number of reports of objective improvements in the course of labour from Malcovati in Italy, Jiminez in Madrid, de Watteville in Switzerland and Trampuz in Yugoslavia, but we have not been able to check the original papers. Lamaze *et al.* (1954) were content to classify results on their own scales of success 'based on the behaviour of the woman as observed by her attendants and on their account as labour proceeds, and also on the objective elements of the perception of uterine activities'. Their course of preparation consisted of nine classes, three on labour given by doctors (one being a psychiatrist) and six by physiotherapists. The results of 863 confinements were as follows: 'Excellent 30.%, Très Bien 18.6%, Bien 21.6%, Mediocre 25.1% and Chec 4.3%'.

There have, however, been two recent studies, one from Australia and the other from Canada, which appear to have been carefully controlled. Sharley (1970) in South Australia compared 600 trained with 600 untrained women matched for parity and age. The training was carefully described and appeared to follow the Lamaze method closely but it included 'reassurance that the acceptance of drugs was not a criterion of failure'. Results showed that the trained group had shorter labours, less anaesthesia, more intact perineums and the Apgar rating of the babies was higher.

The study from Canada was reported by Murray Enkin at an international conference in London in 1971. It is particularly interesting because, owing to lack of accommodation, it was possible to include in the study one group of patients who had requested but been refused training. Three groups, each of 28 mothers, were matched for age, parity, and 'level of education', the classes programme was modelled on that advocated by the American Society for Psychoprophylaxis in Obstetrics, and husbands and wives attended together. Patients who took classes required less sedation, less anaesthesia and less operative intervention than either of the other groups. They reported significantly more favourable experiences in labour and delivery than the controls.

Further good results from the University of Tubingen in Germany were described by Conradt *et al.* at the 4th International Congress of Psychosomatic Medicine in Obstetrics and Gynaecology in Tel Aviv in 1974. Reporting to the International Congress of Psychosomatic Obstetrics and Gynaecology in Rome in 1977 Jušnić *et al.* compared the amount of pain reported by two groups of women, 522 trained and 380 untrained. In the prepared group slight pain was noted in 65.33% of women, tolerable pain in 28.73%, and intolerable pain in 5.94%. In the control group 27.63% experienced extremely severe pain, 57.9% tolerable pain and only 14.47% slight pain.

The second subjective criterion for assessment of the results of psychophysical preparation was the patient's attitude during labour. They were judged on their readiness to apply their training and to cooperate with the obstetrical team. 32.9% of the unprepared patients showed lack of discipline and an inadequate attitude during labour, 39.47% had a satisfactory attitude, and 27.63% a very good one, cooperating actively in the course of delivery. In the trained group of patients an inadequate attitude was noted in only 4.41%, an adequate one in 15.71% and a very good one in 79.88%. We are not told how the two groups were matched.

Conradt selected three approximately matched groups out of a total of 1859 women, the first group were fully prepared by the 'Read method', the second by a short talk and demonstration at the time of admission and the third were unprepared. He found that the women in the first two groups had more rapid dilatation but a slightly slower second stage. The Apgar score of the babies was higher in spite of the fact that all groups were given the same amount of pethidine and the percentage of breast fed babies was also higher.

In America, in 1975, Susan Doering and Doris Entwisle compared 269 women who had been matched with a similar number trained in an intensive course of 'psychoprophylaxis'. The ones who had not had the course were divided into three 'levels'—level one 'did not want to know anything', level two had read books about pregnancy, and level three had done some relaxation.

It is common in America to be highly medicated, almost to general anaesthesia, for the birth, and the first group had 84% fully conscious and only 5% unconscious, while level one of the second group had only 37% remaining partly conscious. Level two (knowledge only) had 69% partly conscious, though only 4% remained conscious and aware throughout labour.

Interviewed afterwards, the more aware the women remained, the more positive and good feelings were retained about childbirth. Ninety-one per cent of those who remained conscious felt positively about the experience, while only 3% of the sedated mothers had a positive feeling about labour. More importantly, perhaps, 59% of the unconscious women had an initial negative reaction to their babies, while the first group registered an 8% negative reaction initially.

When the mothers with a positive attitude were questioned about breast feeding, 59% had breast fed for more than six months, compared to 20% of the mothers with initial negative attitudes. 51% of the 'negative' mothers did not even begin to breast feed.

In America, in 1977, R. J. Stevens and F. Heide did a 'pain trial' of women after various degrees of relaxation training. The experiment was to immerse a hand in ice-water for as long as possible, then warm it to blood heat, and immerse it again, four times. The results were that the ones who had received the least training tolerated the iced water for the shortest times, and repeat immersions became shorter. The ones with the most intensive training tolerated the iced water for much the longest times, and, interestingly, with each new immersion, their tolerance level was increased.

The length and concentration of the training, Stevens and Heide concluded, were as important as the motivation and personalities of the people who attend classes.

Some other evidence also suggests that we are using the right techniques to combat pain and stress. McCaul et al (1979) investigated the 'Effects of paced respirations on psychological and physiological responses to threat'. While waiting to receive electric shocks 105 males either (a) regulated their breathing at half the normal rate (b) regulated their breathing at the normal rate or (c) did not regulate their breathing. Half of the subjects in each group were told that their breathing task would aid them to relax whereas the other half were not given this expectation. Subjects in a no threat condition were not threatened with shocks, did not regulate breathing and were not provided with expectations.

The results indicated that slowing the respiratory rate reduced physiological arousal as measured by skin resistance and finger pulse volume (but not heart rate) and reduced self-reports of anxiety. The authors suggest that their data provide evidence for the effectiveness of paced respiration as a coping strategy, and that they resolve the conflicting findings of previous investigations.

Conclusions. Although there are now a number of centres in this country where psychoprophylaxis, or at least a good psychological and physical training programme, is in force, and where obstetricians take an active part in the preparation programme and mothers are encouraged to put into practice in labour what they have learned in class, we know of no large-scale survey which has been published recently. One is therefore left with no consensus of opinion about the value of preparation on labour. The reasons for the marked differences in results here and abroad are interesting. Are our principles of evaluation stricter, or is the quality of our classes poorer; is our general obstetric care better so that classes have less impact, or is it a question of the interaction of the personalities of those who come to classes with those who teach, support and deliver them?

The value of the group

Many people believe that group therapy is one of the most valuable aspects of classes for expectant mothers and this view was confirmed by the Royal College of Midwives survey (1966 p. 47). Of a sample of 951 mothers, 64% said that the thing they liked best about the classes was the opportunity to 'attend with other expectant mothers'. The value of group discussion in changing attitudes was demonstrated by Friedman in 1971. The 130 women who 'voluntarily expressed the desire for natural childbirth' were interviewed by him at the beginning and end of the course to determine their motivation. He classed such factors as 'strong desire to participate actively for the sheer joy of motherhood' and similar attitudes as positive, and fears and anxieties relating to potential harm during childbirth as negative, and found that 'the training program had altered the importance of the motivating factors from an almost equal distribution at the first interview, to a preponderance of positive over negative factors at the second'.

Preparing for the baby

In the RCM survey (1966) between 40 and 50% of each sample said that they found instruction in bathing, feeding and planning for the baby very helpful, although there were criticisms that the subject of the layette was taken too late in the course. A surprisingly high number (41%) did not find talk on the emotional needs of the baby helpful (p. 46).

Chamberlain and Chave (1977) published an interesting study on the value of different forms of antenatal instruction by comparing 1226 women's reactions to group talks, questions in the antenatal clinics, reading and watching or listening to radio and television broadcasts. Forty-nine per cent of the women, of whom 90% were primiparae, including a number from social class V, attended the talks; three-quarters of them said they had found the talks interesting but only half of them said they had learned anything. Requests were made for the inclusion of practical relaxation and breathing training which were not included in the talks. Three-quarters of the respondents said that they had had adequate opportunities for asking questions at the antenatal clinics. Some found the answers more useful than the talks though there was criticism about lack of time and privacy and the continual changes of doctors. Four-fifths of all the patients said that they had read something about motherhood and child care, mostly the booklet provided by the clinic. The authors remark that 'although the great majority of the patients had made use of published material in preparing themselves for motherhood, there was no indication whatever from this enquiry that their reading could provide a substitute for personal teaching at the clinic. Rather it was looked upon as supplementary to it'. About one-fifth of all the mothers had watched an appropriate programme on television or listened to a radio broadcast.

After the women in the antenatal sample had delivered they were sent a follow-up questionnaire. The authors were disappointed to discover that as many as one-third of the women who had been to the talks found them of no real help in their time of need. Comments here included such remarks as 'Too little was said about the emotional and psychological aspects of pregnancy, we should have been told more about epidurals and what to expect in the lying-in period'.

There is considerable evidence from such organisations as the La Leche League and the Breast Feeding Promotion Group of the National Childbirth Trust that there is a strong association between both pre- and postnatal support and successful breast feeding. The RCM survey sounds a note of warning that during discussion parents 'frequently expressed concern about what they interpreted as their lecturer's strong bias in favour of breast feeding' and their feeling that they would be considered uncooperative or inadequate if they did not conform (p. 46).

Classes for husbands

The evidence of the value of antenatal education to husbands, either through their wives or directly by attendance at classes, is very scanty. In 1966 only 16% of the RCM survey's total sample were invited to fathers' classes. This situation has undoubtedly changed during the last few years and it is now common practice to include at least one fathers' evening in most courses and the number of joint husband and wife courses is growing. According to this survey 54% of the husbands were said to show very great interest and a further 3% some interest in their wives' classes.

Pawson and Morris (1971) reported a study of 730 husbands who attended the two instruction film and discussion sessions as part of the course in psychoprophylaxis at Charing Cross Hospital. The social grouping of these men showed a very strong bias to the upper groups. It was noted that 61.3% of them were present for the whole of labour, 34.4% of these were upset by some aspect of labour, but their presence was considered to be helpful by 92% of all the husbands who attended the labours. They gave the following reasons: raising their wife's morale, improving her physical comfort, helping her to carry out her training, and noting an improvement in their relationship with their wives.

Negative results

It seems that the value of good antenatal education is now proven, though in the Chamberlain survey the type given only helped two-thirds of the women. There is no direct evidence of the harm that unwise teaching can do, but many people will describe adverse behaviour that may well result from it.

Although a lack of enthusiasm in the teacher will lead to badly attended, uninteresting classes where little will be absorbed, over-enthusiasm, and a glowing, unrealistic presentation of labour, offering more than can be achieved, will lead mothers to expect too much of themselves. Too rigid or too didactic teaching may cause a woman to feel that she *must* breathe in a particular pattern, or that her labour will inevitably take a particular form. Thus a woman may try too hard to achieve specific breathing, or be unpleasantly surprised by many aspects of her labour. To quote Buckley (1977) 'to say that labour and delivery will follow a cookbook type of schedule only places the patient in jeopardy of losing all benefits of training when irregularities occur. When a single teacher faces the patients of many doctors there is no way in which all possible occurrences can be encompassed in the classes. A more realistic approach would be to allow for the unknown variables and to condition the patients to handle them as necessary should they occur.'

Recently Docherty & Leather (1982) have taken up this challenge in Scotland with an interesting project. They have prepared a booklet for antenatal mothers in high risk groups aimed at a reading age of 12 years. They have tested its acceptability as to content, style and language by discussion with numerous groups of these mothers and are now experimenting with its effects when freely issued.

Reality means emphasising hard work and concentration, and never giving suggestions of 'painlessness' but painting true pictures on as large a canvas as possible. We ourselves would never wish to talk of 'success' or 'failure', except the success of complete teamwork which includes the parents as members of the obstetric team, and results in a healthy and happy mother and child.

To summarise, one of the great challenges to the future of antenatal education is to make classes so real, interesting and relevant to all socio-economic groups that the attendance is no longer mainly from social classes I to III but is a total cross-section of childbearing women.

REFERENCES

Buckley, D. (1977) Iatrogenic stress in prepared childbirth. In 5th International Congress of Psychosomatic Obstetrics & Gynaecology, vol 20B, pp 901–903. London: Academic Press

Burnett, C W. F. (1956) The value of antenatal exercises. Journal of Obstetrics and Gynaecology of the British Empire, 63, 40.

Chamberlain, G. & Chave, S. (1977) Antenatal education. Community Healh, 9.(1) 12–15.

Chertok, L. (1959) Psychosomatic Methods in Painless Childbirth. Oxford: Pergamon.

Conradt, A., Schlotter, C., Unbehavn, V., Frick, V. & Welsh, P. (1974) Proceedings of the 4th International Congress of Psychosomatic Medicine in Obstetrics and Gynaecology. Basel: Karger. p. 347–350.

Dochery, S. & Leather, D. (1982) Antenatal and child care education—a Scottish response. Health Education Journal, 41, 3

Doering, S. G. & Entwisle, D. R. (1975) Preparation during pregnancy and ability to cope with labour and delivery. American Journal of Orthopsychiatry, 45, 825–37.

Ebner, M. (1973) A Way to Natural Childbirth, 4th edn. Edinburgh: Churchill Livingstone.

Enkin, M. W., Smith, S., Dermer, S. & Emmett, J. (1971) An adequately controlled study of the effectiveness of P. P. M. training. In Third International Congress of Psychosomatic Medicine in Obstetrics and Gynaecology, p. 62. Basel: Karger.

Friedman, D. D. (1971) Motivation for natural childbirth. In Third International Congress of Psychosomatic Medicine in Obstetrics and Gynaecology, p. 30. Basel: Karger.

Harrison, S. (1979) Gynaecological conditions. In *Cash's Textbook of Physiotherapy in some Surgical Conditions*, 6th edn, p. 86. London: Faber & Faber

Huntingford, P. (1965) Objective results of training on labour. In *The Effects of Education for Childbearing on the Mother's Wellbeing*, Conference Report of Obstetric Association of Chartered Physiotherapists, p. 21. Matthews, A. E. and Williams, M. and Odoni.

Južnić, Nh., Vojvodić, L. & Avramović, D. (1977) Psychoprophylaxis today. Evaluation of psychological analgesia during delivery. In *5th International Congress of Psychosomatic Obstetrics & Gynaecology*, vol 20B, pp. 951–954. London: Academic Press

Lamaze, F., Vellay, P., Hersilie, H., Angelergues, H. & Bourrel, A. (1954) Experience pratiqué à la Maternité du Centre Pierre Rouques sur la méthode d'accouchement sans douleur par la psychoprophylaxie. *Bulletin de l'Académie de médecine*, **138**, 52.

McCaul, K., Solomon, S. & Holmes, D. (1979) Effects of paced respiration and expectations on physiological and psychological responses to threat. *Journal of Personality and Social Psychology*, **37**, 4, 564.

Mandelstam, D. (1971) The value of antenatal preparation—a statistical survey. *Midwife and Health Visitor*, 7(6), 217.

Mantle, M., Greenwood, R. & Currey, H. (1977) Backache in pregnancy. *Rheumatology & Rehabilitation*, **16**, 95.

Mantle, M., Holmes, J. & Currey, H. (1981) Backache in pregnancy II Prophylactic influence of back care classes. *Rheumatology & Rehabilitation*, **20**, 227–232.

Matthews, A. E. W. (1965) Subjective results of training for labour. In *Effects of Education for Childbearing on the Mother's Wellbeing*, Conference Report of Obstetric Association of Chartered Physiotherapists, p. 27. Obtainable from Mrs G. Culverwell, M.C.S.P., 40. Days Lane, Biddenham, Bedford

Pawson, M. & Morris, N. (1971) The role of the father in pregnancy and labour. In *Third International Congress of Psychosomatic Medicine in Obstetrics and Gynaecology*, p. 271. Basel: Karger.

Peel, J. H. (1955) Physiotherapy and antenatal care. *Physiotherapy*, **41**(4), 105.

Rathbone, B. (1973) *Focus on New Mothers*. London: Royal College of Nursing.

Roberts, H., Wooten, L., Kane, K. & Harnett, W. (1953) The value of antenatal preparation. *Journal of Obstetrics and Gynaecology of the British Empire*, **60**, 404.

Royal College of Midwives (1966) *Preparation for Parenthood*. Taunton: Barnicotts.

Sharley, C. (1970) The value of physiotherapy in obstetrics. *Medical Journal of Australia*, **6**, 1159.

Stevens, R. J. & Heide, F. (1977) Analgesic characteristics of prepared childbirth techniques; attention focussing and systemic relaxation. *Journal of Psychomatic Research*, **21**, 429–438.

For further evidence of the value of pelvic floor exercise see:

Shepherd, A., Montgomery, E. (1983) Treatment of genuine stress incontinence with a new perineometer. *Physiotherapy*, **69**; 4, 113.

Stoddart, G. (1983) Research project into the effect of pelvic floor exercises on genuine stress incontinence. *Physiotherapy*, **69**, 5, 148–149.

Appendix

Films, filmstrips, slides and useful addresses in the United Kingdom and overseas

(New material at date of publication marked by asterisk*).

FILMS

Pregnancy and birth

Barnet (The Child) 16 mm Sound, Colour, Three films with English commentary, each approximately 20 minutes in length, covering (1) Conception (2) Pregnancy (3) Birth.

These Swedish films cover the whole story of conception, pregnancy and birth using the story of a young couple having their first baby. There are points of difference from the British methods of delivery but the husband—wife sequences are delightful.
Available for hire from National Audio Visual Aids Library, 2 Paxton Place, Gipsy Road, London S.E. 27.

Ready for Baby 16 mm Sound, Colour, 23 minutes
Traces preparation classes by various members of the hospital staff for a group of Irish mothers, and shows several of them in the first and second stages of labour. One mother is delivered on her side, another on her back, with a drip in her arm. In each case the baby is filmed from the mother's angle and is joyfully welcomed. No fathers are present.
Not available for hire. Can be bought from Glaxo Laboratories Ltd, Greenford, Middlesex.

The First Days of Life 16 mm Sound, Colour, 22 minutes
This film begins rather startlingly with a French doctor exhorting a mother to push in second stage. By the time the baby is born, a few minutes later, to the doctor's 'Doucement, doucement' one could begin to wonder about translation problems. However, at this point, an English voice says 'This is not the first day of life', and the rest of the film has clear photographs of the growth of the fetus from

ovum to birth. We see the child growing from a cluster of cells, the buds of the limbs forming, the free movement in mid-pregnancy, thumb-sucking *in utero*, and much more. The film ends almost as it began—the last few minutes goes back to the birth, and the fade-out shots are of a family going off to the beach.

This is not a new film, and each time it is shown, husbands show great interest. Wives report that their husbands suddenly begin to believe in the baby as a person.

Available from the National Audio-Visual Aids Library, 2 Paxton Place, Gipsy Road, London S.E.27.

Family Matters Taken from 'Facts of Life Series', Granada Television.
Four films, starting from early pregnancy to one-year-old. Each part, 16 mm Sound, Colour, 20 minutes.
1. Pregnancy
2. Antenatal classes and birth.
3. Home deliveries, forceps, Caesarian section, breast and bottle feeding.
4. The needs of the new baby. Birth to one year of age.
Available for sale or hire from Concord Films Council Ltd, 201 Felixstowe Road, Ipswich, Suffolk.

The Waiting Game 16 mm Sound, Colour, 33 minutes*
This shows three couples talking about their anxieties, restrictions, discomforts, relationships during late pregnancy, followed by the births of their babies. They are all primiparae, adjusting to this new experience. A sympathetic doctor discusses induction. An ultra-sound scan is shown. Each birth starts differently, but only in one birth is much of the first stage shown (here the couple were not given correct advice on the telephone, and had not packed a case). There are discussion points throughout the film.

One birth was induced—the 'drip' is shown. One had a forceps delivery—focus on mother's face, not on the forceps. Pain mentioned frequently, and all second stages looked, not only tremendously hard work, but painful.

There is great involvement by all three husbands in the labour, and the emotional scenes after the births are very moving. However, in each case, the baby was held by the parents for a very brief time before being removed for weighing, etc., and none of the mothers breastfed immediately.

For maximum reality, there has been some loss of sound quality.

It is advised to turn up tenor sounds, and turn down base, if this is possible on the projector. Otherwise, the projectionist can adjust the sound to different speech as the film runs.

The film needs a good introduction, and time for discussion afterwards. Excellent to be shown to fathers, and also useful for any professionals in contact with expectant parents.

Available for purchase or hire from Farley's Health Products, Film Library, Torr Lane, Plymouth.

A Child is Born 16 mm Sound, Colour, 20 minutes★

Made in France, this is a film made to show Dr Leboyer's methods of gentle childbirth. Dr Leboyer himself conducts the delivery, and he, as well as the mother, strokes the baby. The baby looks calm and alert. This is a good teaching aid for those who would like to learn the techniques from the originator himself.

Available for sale or hire from Guild Sound and Vision, 82–129 Oundle Road, Peterborough.

Your Baby's Birth 16 mm Sound, Colour, 20 minutes★

This is mainly about normal labour, but there are short explanations and pictures of an induction, epidural analgesia, forceps, breech and a Caesarian section. Fathers are shown giving great help and support. The delivery scenes are realistic 'bottom of the bed' pictures, and may possibly make some expectant mothers apprehensive. This film *must* be known by the person showing it, so that she can introduce it well and be ready for questions afterwards.

Available for sale or hire from Sylvia Meredith, Audio-Visual, Health Education Advisory Service, 3 Elgin Road, Sutton, Surrey.

Have a Healthy Baby. Two films:

1. *Pregnancy* 16 mm, Sound, Colour, 22 minutes

   This film examines the physical changes of pregnancy, and the mother's feelings. It stresses the importance of early antenatal care, good nutrition, and exercise.

2. *Labour and Delivery.* 16 mm, Sound, Colour, 29 minutes

   The second part follows two couples through labour and birth. One has a normal labour, the other is more difficult. In both, the father's support is shown to be of great importance for the mother's well-being.

Made in U.S.A. by Churchill Films..

For hire from Concord Film Council, 201 Felixtowe Road, Ipswich, Suffolk.

For sale from Boulton-Hawker Films Ltd., Hadley, Ipswich, Suffolk.

Life Before Birth 16 mm, Sound, Colour, 16 minutes.
This film, made at Queen Charlotte's Hospital, uses pictures of normal human fetuses in normal pregnancies to show the growth and development of the baby in the uterus. It shows intra-uterine life as a busy time for the fetus, and the speed of the changes gives added incentive to the mother to look after herself and her fast-developing baby.
For hire from The Institute of Obstetrics and Gynaecology, Queen Charlotte's Hospital, Goldhawk Road, London, W.6.

It's Not an Illness. 16 mm, Sound, Colour, 24 minutes.
A Canadian film showing normal pregnancy and childbirth. Exercise and positive health and fitness are stressed, also 'natural childbirth.'
For hire from Pegasus Films, 5 Sycamore Villas, West View, Mold, Clwyd, North Wales.

Pregnancy and Childbirth Series. All are 16 mm, Sound, Colour,

Before Pregnancy (8½ minutes)
The importance of good health and the need for parents to have a positive attitude and a willingness to accept the responsibilities of parenthood. Diet, health checks, exercise, and what to avoid in the preconception period.

Prenatal (20 minutes)
The above points again, also the developing baby and antenatal exercises.

Labour and Delivery (18 minutes)
A birth film with the husband helping throughout. It shows an episiotomy, and some problems of the time immediately after birth.

Special Cases (12 minutes)
Caesarean section, forceps delivery, induced labour, epidural anaesthesia.
From Guild Sound and Vision Ltd., 85–129 Oundle Road, Peterborough.

Every Day a Birthday. 16 mm, Sound, Colour, 15 minutes
The events of labour and what happens afterwards up to the time the mother goes home. Most of the film is labour—a normal delivery, epidural analgesia, and a forceps delivery. It was made to familiarise

parents with labour ward situations, but, as we know, these are different to some extent in different places, as each hospital is individual.

For sale or hire from Three Arrows Film Productions, 17 Convent Walk, Sheffield, South Yorkshire.

'Trigger' films (To promote group discussion)*

Having a Baby (All are 16 mm, Sound, Colour, Film or Video)
1. *Lorraine's Story* (7 minutes)
To be shown early in pregnancy with the object of discussing the importance of antenatal care. It is Lorraine's second baby, and she visits her doctor.
2. *Sue's Story* (9 minutes)
Sue visits the antenatal clinic, and later, with her husband, begins to attend antenatal classes. The partner's role in preparation for birth is discussed.
3. *Richard's Story* (7 minutes)
He describes his feelings when he is present at the induced birth of his daughter. The film shows positive ways in which fathers can contribute during labour and delivery.
4. *Eileen and Jan's Stories* (11 minutes)
Eileen had a relaxed and normal first stage, then the cord prolapsed, and an immediate Caesarian section was necessary. The delivery is not shown, but Eileen talks about her memory of events. Jan has a normal delivery and describes her emotions while the birth is being shown. Both the labours focus on the feelings of the parents.
5. *Caroline and John's Story* (8 minutes)
After the baby is born. Both parents talk about the care of their second daughter, and the interaction between the baby and her sister. Breast feeding, fatigue and the father's role are discussed and shown.

Free loan from Concord Films Council Ltd., 201 Felixstowe Road, Ipswich.

For sale from the Supplies Department, Health Education Council, 78 New Oxford Street, London, W.C.1.

The BBC will supply a catalogue of Health and Social Studies Films and Video-Cassettes on request. The catalogue can be obtained from BBC Enterprises, British Broadcasting Corporation, Villiers House, The Broadway, London W.5.

As video-recorders are becoming readily available, the catalogue contains films and video-cassettes. The latter can be bought but not hired.

One set of these video-cassettes, is the series, *Parents and Children—Having a Baby*. There were 16 programmes introduced by Claire Rayner. All are available to be sold separately. Some subjects covered (the catalogue will indicate the topics on each video-cassette) are conception, hospital booking, physiotherapists, health visitors, baby's development, breast and bottle feeding, childbirth, breech birth, AID, special care units, Caesarians, inductions the first weeks of life, the crying baby, and safety in the home.

To describe one video-tape briefly:

This one is *The Birth* Sound, Colour, 25 minutes

It shows the start of labour with backache followed by contractions. A vaginal examination is performed and the mother is made comfortable in the first stage room, which contains a rocking chair. Breathing through contractions is juxtaposed with animated diagrams of the first stage process.

A pethidine injection is given. When second stage begins, again good animated diagrams show what is happening. Gas and oxygen is used at the beginning of contractions, then the mother gets into a comfortable pushing position. The midwife encourages her, and her partner supports her head.

Between contractions, he makes her comfortable and mops her face. During contractions, he counts the seconds as she holds her breath. An episiotomy is shown, discreetly. A good delivery is followed by the baby being quickly wrapped and handed to the parents. The placenta is delivered and the baby examined. Stitches are inserted while the father is present. Breast feeding, with the baby sucking well, is followed by a cup of tea for the parents. A detailed paediatric examination is carried out on the fifth day, with the mother involved. The paediatrician explains the primary reflexes to her as he demonstrates them, and assures her that the baby is fine, and can focus on her face when she is feeding. Questions are answered.

There are 15 films, each lasting 25 minutes. The catalogue is updated regularly. We see video-cassettes being one of the major educational media of the present generation.

Address

To purchase only.
(Films and Video-Cassettes).

BBC Enterprises Film and Video Sales.
Villiers House
The Broadway
London, W.5.

The newborn, the growing baby and the family

Child Development in the First Year 16 mm Sound, Colour, 30 minutes. Long and delightful sequences of the spontaneous behaviour of infants. The film shows clearly the basic milestones of development. It seeks to show how much can be learnt about the general progress of a baby, in gross and fine motor movements and in communication, from observation of his behaviour in play situations.
From Camera Talks, 31 North Row, London W.1. For sale or hire.

The Amazing Newborn 16 mm Sound, Colour, 35 minutes*
This begins with the birth of a baby, then his serene mother holding him. The film demonstrates that a baby, from birth, is a responsive, reacting, learning child. Infants of under seven days are shown reacting to the human voice, to touch, to eye contact, to light.

Part of the film is slowed down, showing the babies moving their limbs to the rhythm of their mothers' voices.

With a gentle, normal delivery, the child's first hour is spent in quiet alertness, so that at birth he is ready for bonding, and should be allowed this relaxed time in his mother's arms.

Three sleep stages are identified—quiet sleep, R.E.M. (rapid eye movement) sleep, and drowsiness. Then the baby's learning and responding ability is reached. A crying baby changes in the film to a quiet, alert baby when held closely, and, in his mother's arms, this is a time to learn and communicate. The baby is shown actively doing this in his first few days of life.

The whole film shows the infant as participating in interpersonal relationships from birth, and the babies are photographed beautifully and with great skill. The film could perhaps make parents anxious to elicit the same responses from their newly-born children, and not succeed as well as shown here. Certainly, anyone seeing this film would not expect a baby simply to 'sleep and feed' and would be more aware of the baby as a personality.
Available for sale or hire from the Health Services Communication Center, Cleveland, Ohio.

With a Little Help 16 mm Sound, Colour, 35 minutes⋆
This film is meant to follow *The Waiting Game* and it was intended to show the same three couples in the post partum period. One couple had moved, so a new couple is introduced.

Again, this has been designed to promote discussion, and this time to show the reality of the first days with a new baby. Some expectant parents have criticised it as it tends to show more of the problems than the joys of parenthood—but parents of second or subsequent babies have welcomed the film as being much nearer the truth than the glossy advertisements of motherhood.

In this hospital, discharge of mother and baby is early, and therefore, the midwife visits at home until at least the tenth day. Her role in teaching and helping the parents is shown—especially when she is called out at night to a fretful baby and very anxious parents.

Parents' swings of mood are made clear—the father's loneliness when his wife is in hospital, and again his isolation when his wife is spending her evenings upstairs with the baby. Postnatal 'blues' are photographed and discussed very naturally, as is night tiredness and tension. A supporting granny and an unhelpful granny are introduced with tact, as is also the father's support and his need to be drawn into helping with the baby. The health visitor is shown as someone who advises with sympathy and good sense, rather than actively doing things for the baby. She is shown discussing rest, postnatal exercises, family planning, etc.

The complete change in life style is emphasised.

(See note on sound in *The Waiting Game*).

Available for sale or hire from Farley's Health Products, as before.

Breast Feeding—A Special Closeness 16 mm Sound, Colour, 30 min⋆
A comprehensive film, very well photographed, starting with advice on the care and preparation of the breasts in pregnancy. Shows successful breast feeding looking easy and comfortable, including casual breast feeding in unusual places, proving that modesty can be maintained, for instance, at choir practice and in the park. Discussion of demand feeding, breast feeding after a Caesarian section, sibling reaction, and complications, with solutions. Also shows it is possible to go back to work, express and store milk, and talks of the benefits of breast feeding.

A teaching guide is supplied, with discussion topics and bibliography.

Only obtainable from the U.S.A. at the moment, from Motion Inc., 4437 Kingle Street, N.W., Washington DC 20016.

Understanding Breast Feeding 16 mm Sound, Colour, 25 minutes★
This is a factual film, describing the anatomy and physiology of the breast, and the mechanics of breast feeding. There are many details about breast preparation, 'fixing' the baby correctly on the areolar tissue, and dealing with difficulties such as engorgement. Although the film gives lots of information, there is very little emotion, and problems seem to be emphasised. The pleasure of breast feeding is not mentioned.
Available for sale or hire from Farley's Health Products, Film Library, Torr Lane, Plymouth.

Mother's Own 16 mm Sound, Colour, 25 minutes★
This film begins with the baby's birth, then follows with a series of mothers describing the experience of breast feeding their babies, and at times the lack of help they received from hospital staff.
Hire only from Concord Film Company Ltd, 201 Felixstowe Road, Ipswich.

The Bond of Breast Feeding 16 mm Sound, Colour, 20 minutes★
By contrast to the last film, this presents the facts of breast feeding in a very positive and quite emotional manner. It is much more a film about feelings and closeness. Although most of the mothers are American, perhaps members of the La Leche League when considering some of their statements, it was made in England, and the narrator is Dr Hugh Jolly. (The La Leche League is an American organisation to promote breast feeding—there is now a branch in England.)

Very relaxed, rather upper-class mothers are shown, and the photography is beautiful. Eye-to-eye contact between mother and infant is emphasised, and the film begins with a newborn baby being stroked by the mother and gently put to the breast, when contented sucking begins immediately. Comments have been that this is slightly idealistic, and, indeed, the whole film has a pleasure emphasis, for both mother and baby, although early difficulties are mentioned. Fathers are included, and the breast feeding is seen as adding to family closeness.

For mothers who really want to feed, and are successful, this is an ideal film. Multigravidae who have enjoyed their first experience have said it 'brought it all back'.

Reservations would be the effect the film may have on people who definitely want to bottle feed, or those who want to breast feed and fail to do so. May they perhaps remember statements such as 'Lactation is the fourth part of pregnancy' or 'The intensity helps

the bonding process'? We can see that for some groups, therefore *Understanding Breast Feeding* may be more acceptable, but this is a lovely film.
Available for sale or hire from Metromed, Metropolis House, Neals Yard, Covent Garden, London W.C.2.

Breast Feeding 16 mm, Sound, Colour, 20 minutes
Made by S.M.A. baby foods, this film opens with a group of mothers who give what sound like very acceptable reasons for either failing to continue or never starting to breast feed their babies. A paediatrician then stresses the value of breast feeding and there are attractive pictures of mothers nursing their babies. One is left with the impression that failure to persevere with breast feeding does not matter very much as long as the right product is substituted.
Obtainable from John Wyeth & Brother Ltd, Taplow, Maidenhead, Berks.

Hello Baby 16 mm Sound, Colour, 25 minutes*
This film is an award-winner, and has beautiful photography. It films babies in six different families from birth to 15 months, and shows especially how fathers can be actively involved with their children and enjoy their growth, and play, from their earliest days of life. Development is shown through everyday activities. Wide ranges of normal growth and learning are filmed and the help of the health visitor, doctor and clinic is mentioned, especially when the child is thought be developing out of this 'normal' range. A leaflet explaining what development would be expected at six different ages is available with the film.
Free hire from the Central Film Library, Government Buildings, Bromyard Avenue, Acton, London W.3.

Katy's First Year Sound, Colour, 25 minutes*
This film, sponsored by Robinson's Baby Foods, shows a child's progress from her birth to her first birthday. The film was produced, and the linking commentary spoken, by Katy's father, so he obviously does not feature. It is essentially a scrapbook of a mother and her baby, with all other commentary by Dr Hugh Jolly. He is also shown helping Katy's mother to understand Katy's responses and her learning abilities. Perhaps slightly 'up-market', but a very good observational film of actions, reactions, changes and growth. As Katy becomes more mobile, her elder brother's natural periods of annoyance and jealousy are discussed. A guide to the film is provided, and indicates discussion points. A very good film,

especially for mothers and mothers-to-be, but also for all people involved with child care and normal growth.
For sale or hire from Concord Films Council Ltd, 201 Felixstowe Road, Ipswich, Suffolk.

Getting to Know Each Other 16 mm, Sound, Colour, 22 minutes, Film or video★
This and the following film were planned by Dr Aidan MacFarlane, Clinical Lecturer in Paediatrics in Oxford, to illustrate the perception and understanding of newborn infants, and how mothers get to know their babies.

This film, by simple experiments, shows that in the first seven days of life the baby can see, focus, hear, taste, and smell, and can recognise and respond to his mother.

It is an excellent film to make the antenatal mother aware of her baby as a thinking, learning person and to give her a sense of the reality of the baby she is carrying.

Changing Days 16 mm, Sound, Colour, 19 minutes, Film or Video★
Again we concentrate on the baby's first seven days—not with clinical experiments, but with the reactions of mothers and babies to each other. The film shows a primipara learning what her baby needs, and being helped by other mothers who have had babies before and are giving practical guidance.

The mother is portrayed as she gains confidence during these days, and the baby as he responds to this confidence, to her voice, her touch, and her comfort. The support which mothers in hospital get from each other, and the security this brings to both mothers and babies, is well illustrated.
Both films are for hire or sale from Farley Health Products Ltd., Torr Lane, Plymouth, Devon.

And Baby Makes Three 16 mm, Sound, Colour★
This film is divided into two parts, to be shown separately or together.
Part 1. *Baby's View* 9 minutes
A brief montage of two births continues with life from the 'baby's angle'—the cameras attempt to give a vision of the world with the baby's range of focus. It shows breast feeding, crying, playing and stimulation, and the baby's reactions to its environment.
Part 2. *Parents' View* 13 minutes
Again the two births, then the adjustment in the first six weeks

as the couple become a family of three. The parents talk about being overwhelmed by the baby's demands at first, and their need of reor-ganisation. The importance of getting out, of seeing friends, and of the husband's help in coping with changes in their home life, are all illustrated well.

For hire from Random Film Library, 25 The Burroughs, Hendon, London, N.W.4.

Feeding is Loving 16 mm, Sound, Colour, Film or Video★
Beginning from the premise that babies need love, warmth and good food for healthy growth, the film traces infant feeding from birth to nine months, showing the development from breast or bottle to a full mixed diet. The mother's food is discussed, with the main food groups for health illustrated. Then five babies are filmed, at home and in a well-baby clinic. The different needs at each stage of growth are emphasised, and also the importance of play, conversation and affection in the making of a happy, well-nourished child.

Free loan from the Central Film Library, Chalfont Grove, Gerrards Cross, Buckinghamshire.

The Generation Game 16 mm, Sound, Colour, 22 minutes★
Food in the first year of life. This film has the message that infant feeding is not simply a series of do's and dont's. It is fundamentally about developing good nutritional habits for life—and for the next generation.

Couples and families are shown participating in a 'television game', similar to the original 'Generation Game', with all the ques-tions and decisions concentrated on feeding the family, from birth to ordinary family meals.

For hire from Farley Health Products Ltd., Torr Lane, Plymouth, Devon.

Bathing a Baby—A Touch of Love 16 mm, Sound, Colour, 18 minutes★
This film shows how baby's bathtime plays an important role in the bonding process between mother and baby.

For hire from Random Film Library, 25 The Burroughs, London, N.W.4.

From Cradle Days to Family Meals 16 mm, Sound, Colour, 22 minutes★
Teaches correct feeding techniques with breast and bottle. Then

there is a gradual progression from the first breast feed, through weaning, to home cooking
For hire from Eothen Films Ltd., E.M.I. Studios, Shenley Road, Borehamwood, Hertfordshire.

Where Love Ends 16 mm, Sound, Colour, 23 minutes
A teaching film made by Milton Hygiene, showing everyday routines such as bottle feeding and the sterilising of feeding equipment, bathing, napkin-changing, and napkin hygiene. It emphasises that if a mother starts with a good routine it will become automatic, and ensure high standards of safety for the baby in the home.
For sale or hire from Guild Sound and Vision Ltd., Woodston House, Oundle Road, Peterborough.

Baby in the House Sound, Colour, 20 minutes*
The film depicts two situations which are fairly true to life. In the first, a young, over-anxious mother attempts unsuccessfully to make her baby conform to her routine, and is helped by her health visitor to modify her life-style to cope with the baby more happily.

In the second situation an older, experienced mother is advised to bottle feed by her doctor. She has not bottle-fed before, and experiences difficulties which are resolved with the help of her midwife.
For hire from The Film Librarian, Wyeth Laboratories, Taplow, Maidenhead, Buckinghamshire.

Family planning

Happy Family Planning 16 mm Music, Colour, 10 minutes
This brief cartoon film shows present methods of birth control in a clear, easily assimilated and amusing fashion. There is a musical background, but no speech. Its great advantage, for a multiracial audience especially, is that it has captions in several languages, including Urdu, but is clear enough to be understood without reading ability.
It can be hired from the Concord Films Council, 201 Felixstowe Road, Ipswich.

Every Baby a Wanted Baby 16 mm Sound, Colour, 35 minutes
This begins with a lecture at a family planning clinic, with diagrams of male and female reproductive systems and fertilisation. It goes on

to show clearly each type of birth control at present in use, and evaluates each method. As it was made in 1968, there is perhaps more emphasis on the sheath and diaphragm cap than on contraceptive pills and intrauterine devices. It accepts that religious conviction may influence the choice of family planning methods, and emphasises the importance of individual preferences.

Available on free loan from L. R. Industries Ltd, Hall Lane, London E.4.

If wished, L. R. Industries will supply a projector, and a projectionist who is prepared to answer questions.

Methods of Family Planning 16 mm Sound, Colour, 20 minutes
This begins with a description of the male and female anatomy, and the reproductive process; then in a Family Planning Clinic setting, it discusses with several different couples all known recommended methods of contraception.

Sale or hire from Concord Film Company Ltd, 201 Felixstowe Road, Ipswich.

Contraceptives 16 mm, Sound, Colour, 23 minutes*
International Planned Parenthood Film, available in Arabic, French, Spanish or English.

All methods of contraception are explained in an acceptable way for non-medical viewers.

English version for hire from Concord Films Council, 201, Felixstowe Road, Ipswich, Suffolk.

Other languages—for sale only, from The International Planned Parenthood Federation, 18–20. Lower Regent Street, London, S.W.1. (Catalogue available of a series of films on family planning in different languages. Address as above).

New Relations 16 mm, Sound, Colour, 34 minutes*
Made in the U.S.A., this film features a father exploring the costs—both financial and emotional—of having decided to become a father. He also considers the rewards, especially of choosing to share child care responsibilities equally with his wife, who also has a career. Together, they plan to wait a little longer before another child is born.

For hire from Concord Films Council Ltd., 201 Felixstowe Road, Ipswich, Suffolk.

Trigger Film. To Plan your Family 16 mm, Sound, Colour, 10 minutes*
An animated film, with a description of a woman's reproductive system and the most common methods of contraception. The film should be easy to understand by people of all levels of education.
For hire from Boulton-Hawkes Films Ltd., Hadleigh, Ipswich, Suffolk.

FOR TEACHERS

The Foetus 16 mm Sound, Colour, 25 minutes
Made at Queen Charlotte's Hospital, London, this film shows and discusses all the fetal monitoring we have been mentioning (a very clear example of taking blood from the fetal scalp, with diagrams, is included). Not suitable for pregnant women, but it would help to keep a teacher up to date with recent techniques. Basically, it shows that the fetus and its well-being are not as hidden from us in pregnancy as they were a few years ago.
Can be hired from the British Medical Association Film Library, British Medical Association, BMA House, Tavistock Square, London W.C.1.

Abortion—The Counselling Approach 16 mm Sound, Colour, 29 minutes*
This film concerns counselling about abortion, with two women who have problem pregnancies and need to decide their course of action.
One decides to abort, the other to continue her pregnancy. However, the main purpose of the film is to show the development of the counselling process and human relationships.
Available for sale or hire from Concord Films Council Ltd, 201 Felixstowe Road, Ipswich, Suffolk.

Survival of The Weakest 16 mm Sound, Colour, 45 minutes*
A film to show the advances now being made both in the prevention and the treatment of low birth weight and premature infants. Statistics are given—approximately 50 000 children born each year in the United Kingdom weigh less than 2.5 kg ($5\frac{1}{2}$ lb). The antenatal care in clinics and hospitals is largely designed to pick out mothers and babies who may be 'at risk' for any reason, and to give them good care. Drugs to prevent premature births are mentioned, and the research now going on to achieve even healthier pregnancies, and how we might be able to have many fewer low-weight babies. The film ends on the encouraging note that problems are fewer now, and that there is much more hope for healthier babies.

From BBC Enterprises, U.K. Sale or hire.
Film sales—Villiers House, The Broadway, London, W.5.
Film hire—Woodston House, Oundle Road, Peterborough.
(Plus BBC Enterprises in U.S.A., Canada, South Africa, Australia and New Zealand).

A Question of Confidence 16 mm, Sound, Colour, 30 minutes*
Following the discussions about good antenatal care, which aims at increasing the mother's emotional health, this film shows how it can be done.

Three areas of the country are shown.

1. The Sighthill district of Edinburgh, showing continuity of care based on a Health Centre, in an economically disadvantaged area where a large number of mothers are termed 'high-risk'. Ninety five per cent of these mothers now have antenatal care in early pregnancy, with a team of family doctors and midwives working together. A survey has shown that this early care, continuing through pregnancy, has halved the number of low-birth-weight babies, and more than halved perinatal mortality.

2. St George's Hospital, Tooting. An antenatal clinic where women feel that they are individuals, where the children have somewhere to play, and where mothers are encouraged to express their wishes about labour and delivery. The waiting time is as short as possible, but, while waiting, films and videos about labour and child care are shown. (With Caroline Flint.)

3. King's College Hospital, London. At a special clinic for pregnant teenagers, we see the girls getting warm, loving attention. When they feel their social and emotional needs are being met, they are willing to attend and take advice.

For hire from Concord Films Council Ltd., 201 Felixstowe Road, Ipswich, Suffolk.

Active Birth
Part 1, Sound, Colour, Video*

This video film, with Janet Balaskas, was made at the Royal Free Hospital in London. It shows a labouring woman, with the husband and Janet helping her, doing whatever she feels her body wants her to do in labour.

She walks about in the first stage, sways and rocks with contractions, leans on her husband, but is herself in control. In the second stage she is on hands and knees, and as the baby is born there is a close-up of her face, perspiring, tired, but looking joyful and exalted.

Part 2, Sound, Black and White, Video*

The second part is a home birth, with no commentary. All we hear are the mother's comments and her breathing. Again she moves as she wishes, and spends a lot of time on all-fours, with pelvic rocking and swaying. She is supported by Janet Balaskas, by her midwife, and by her husband, but throughout is in command of herself. The film makes no attempt to hide the hard work, and the energy and intensity of the mother's feelings. The black and white filming gives her movements an added focus—the light is dim, and all is centred on the activity of giving birth.

When the baby is born, he is calm and quiet. He is held by his mother and they look into each other's faces. When she baths him gently, his eyes are still focussed on her face.

Both these films, especially the latter, show the profound experience of giving birth. They should be seen by all teachers who wish to encourage active birth in their classes.

For sale or hire from Phrynee Milne, 48, Middle Lane, Epsom, Surrey. European Sales—P.O. Box 14 000, Utrecht 3508 S.B, The Netherlands.

Birth (A film sponsored by the National Childbirth Trust) 16 mm Colour, Sound, 50 minutes

This film was sponsored by the Trust after it had been completed. Some of the views expressed, therefore, are not views necessarily held by all National Childbirth Trust members.

An advertisement was placed in a National newspaper, asking for volunteers to talk about their experiences of birth. Naturally, the opinions, including distress, anger and happiness thus vary widely; from those who wanted to share a beautiful experience with viewers to those who look back on incidents with horror or indignation. The speakers have vivid recall of events, and although there is some praise of professional services, there are also many comments about actions parents thought of as unnecessary interference or neglect. Between these descriptions, there are regular 'cuts' to the progress of two births, both at home.

Much of the labour is shown in the first delivery, where a comfortable-looking midwife is letting a couple experience labour with very little interference from her. To this mother and father, childbirth is obviously an emotional, sexual, meaningful event in their lives— they feel that they are 'giving birth' together.

The second mother is shown as the baby is being born, a lovely delivery by a Leboyer-trained midwife. The interaction between the parents and the baby, and the calm, interested, wide-eyed face of the baby as he absorbs his immediate surroundings and feelings, is a beautiful thing to watch. Again, it should be seen by all professionals, who will both learn from, and disagree with, many parts of the film. But how can we, as teachers, show this to a group of mothers who are, say, booked for hospital delivery knowing that their care will be different? The contrasting peace of the births, with the comments of the mothers interspersed, is striking, but could be disturbing.

Apply to the NCT, 9 Queensborough Terrace, London, W.2. for hiring details.

Birth—With Dr R. D. Laing 16 mm Sound, Colour, 55 minutes
This is a criticism by a noted psychiatrist on modern delivery techniques: not suitable for a pregnant audience, but it should be seen by every midwife and obstetrician.

Many mothers are interviewed in the film, and almost all their comments are critical—from lack of information to obstetric procedures. The film challenges 'routine' practices, and indeed makes some of them look frightening—showing for instance, a women with legs in the stirrups looking completely helpless, almost crucificial.

The effects on both mother and baby are vividly portrayed—especially the baby's experience of handling and noise, and his terrified cries on being circumcised.

A very good film showing the abuses which Dr Laing feels happen in this period, and making his points extremely strongly.

Leads to controversy when shown to a professional audience. The leader of the discussion should be prepared for this.

Made in New Zealand.

Available for sale or hire from Concord Films Council Ltd, 201 Felixstowe Road, Ipswich, Suffolk and in New Zealand, the New Zealand Arts Council.

Safe and Sound 16 mm Sound, Colour, 43 minutes
The development and value of ultrasonic echo sounding.

Available for sale or hire from Concord Film Company Ltd, 201 Felixstowe Road, Ipswich.

Over to you (Using the overhead projector) 16 mm Sound, Colour, 26 minutes
Although at first this subject does not seem particularly interesting, the film has made it most enjoyable. If an overhead projector is avail-

able for their use, or could be obtained, I would advise any teacher to see this film. It shows the diversity of the projector, and the many ways of using it in teaching. Demonstrations are given of imaginative, colourful ways of producing transparencies, adding overlays and revealing sections at a time until a whole picture is built up. Although the examples do not apply to childbirth, it is obvious in the examples that it could be very easily adapted to antenatal teaching, with fresh bright ideas.

Available for sale or hire from The National Audio-Visual Aids Library, 2 Paxton Place, Gipsy Road, London, S.E.27.

Stillbirth 16 mm Colour, Sound, 12 minutes
A 'must' for all who may be working with bereaved parents, especially doctors and midwives. One woman was interviewed sensitively by Sheila Hancock, who had obvious empathy with her. The mother is a journalist and can express vividly the emotions which other mothers may not be able to vocalise. She talks of the attitudes of people around her—embarrassment, avoidance, a sense of failure—and her own feelings of devastation.

The depth and variety of the emotions include guilt, failure and mourning. She describes them movingly and sincerely.

Stillbirth gives professionals and others help in ways to work with parents suffering this crisis. The film shows the need for explanations, for comfort, listening and understanding, and how cruel it is to dismiss this happening as something a woman will 'get over', and not a real bereavement. To the mother, she has lost a real person, a child she loves.

Available for purchase or hire from Religious Films Ltd, Foundation House, Walton Road, Bushey, Watford.

Feeding Normal Babies 16 mm Sound, Colour, 25 minutes
Part 1 Breast Feeding. Part 2 Bottle Feeding
This film is primarily for midwives and the commentary is directed towards them. Part 1 opens with a technical description of the different constituents of human and cow's milk. The structure and function of the breasts are clearly described and advice given as to their antenatal care. The technique of fixing the baby on the breast and his sucking reflex are shown though there is little evidence of emotional satisfaction to either mother or baby.

Part 2 is a straightforward description of how to prepare and give a bottle feed. There is no obvious propaganda for the manufacturer.
Obtainable from Cow & Gate, Trowbridge, Wiltshire, BA 14 8 HZ

MISCELLANEOUS

An Open University Course made in connection with the BBC and the Health Education Council may be appropriate for those teachers who feel they can get up early to watch television, and be interested in coping with the work sheets, etc.

It is primarily meant for parents who wish to know much more about child development and family interaction. The course lasts eight weeks, and is titled *The First Years of Life*.

At the time of going to press, the Open University is intending to produce the series at regular intervals of under a year. Applications can be made six months before each eight-week session.

It consists, as is usual with OU courses, of television and radio programmes, books to read, charts, work-sheets, leaflets and also three records. Each of the television programmes is available as a video film.

The beginning television programme follows a couple throughout pregnancy and encourages women to ask more questions and know their bodies. The accompanying radio programme has three couples talking about feelings in pregnancy and their fears and expectations.

Then comes a step-by-step guide through birth.

After this, two baby boys, born in the same week, are filmed when eight weeks old, showing their different skills, and what they enjoy and have learned. The radio programme is titled *Down in the Dumps*—a vivid account of the dramatic transformation of one woman's life after the birth of her first baby.

The course continues through the early months and years of life. *More information on the programme times, is available from The Open University, P.O. Box 76, Milton Keynes.*

Facts For Life Series—Family Matters 16 mm or Video, Sound, Colour, 20 minutes each*
A series of eight films made by Granada Television. Education for parenthood, emphasising the child's need for love and security.
1. Conception, fetal growth, antenatal tests
2. Antenatal classes, labour and birth
3. Home and hospital births. Breast and bottle feeding
4. Early development. Health checkups
5. First months of life
6. Development up to four years
7. Care and safety. Immunisation
8. Special needs of children with handicaps.

For hire from Concord Films Council Ltd., 201 Felixstowe Road, Ipswich, Suffolk.

FILMSTRIPS

Pregnancy and birth

The following are all in colour and are standard 35 mm strips or slides.

Your First Baby, Parts 1–3
Part 1: Before. Deals briefly with the early symptoms of pregnancy, suitable food and clothing, Health Service facilities, what to prepare for the baby and how both husband and wife can cope with the varying emotions of pregnancy.

Part 2: During. Gives a detailed account of birth in an ordinary hospital setting. Diagrams and pictures of the three stages of labour, showing two primigravid deliveries, one dorsal, filmed from behind mother's shoulder and the other lateral.

Part 3: After. Deals with the puerperium in hospital and makes some points about coping with the new baby at home, family planning and adjustment to life as a family.

Education for Childbirth, Parts 1–2
Part 1: Psycho-physical preparation. Illustrates how attitudes towards childbirth develop, and shows a class of mothers practising relaxation and breathing with husbands learning to help.

Part 2: Labour. Traces the labour and home delivery of one of these 'prepared' mothers, ably supported by her husband, and ends with the introduction of the new baby to the two little boys. Both strips emphasise the necessary teamwork between the medical attendants taking part and the parents.

Pregnancy—a Challenging Experience, Parts 1 and 2. (See p. 65 for contents.)

Birth—A Shared Experience, Parts 1 and 2
Begins with the story of the birth of a son to one young couple, showing how the husband can help and support his wife in a normal hospital setting. Has attractive shots of the beginning of the parents' bonding with the baby. Other pictures and diagrams illustrate further medical help that may be required in some cases such as induction, fetal monitoring, epidural analgesia, forceps and ventouse extraction.

*Tranquil Delivery**
A delivery filmed at Kings College Hospital, London, showing a modified Leboyer technique. Points illustrated are the mother's position in the second stage, the minimum stimulation of the baby by gentle handling, a quiet and dimly lit delivery room and the maximum skin and eye contact between the parents and the baby. The strip is intended for professionals but by cutting out some of the 'tail-end shots' and modifying the script it could be used for parents.
The above are all available as filmstrips or sets of slides with tapes from Camera Talks, 31 North Row, London, W.1. on a sale or return basis but not for hire.

Baby care

Breast Feeding
Infant Feeding
Clothing Baby
Everyday Care of Your Baby (parents look rather elderly, but this is the fourth child and good teaching points are made)
Safety for Your Baby (from birth to toddler stage)
Child Development in The First Year—Part 1 Large Movements (from sitting to walking)
Part 2 Coordination (from first smile to playing with toys)
All the above available from Camera Talks either as filmstrips or as sets of slides in boxes or in album or cabinet file with or without cassette tape of commentary.

Also available at the present time:
Choosing Baby's Layette
Cold Water Sterilising for Bottles and Teats
Safety in the Home
Baby's Bathtime
All available on free loan from Mrs Sylvia Meredith, Health Education Advisory Service, 3 Elgin Road, Sutton, Surrey (preferably through local health education officers).

Family planning

About Family Planning (A Family Doctor Filmstrip)
A comprehensive filmstrip, beginning with reproduction and unreliable methods of planning, followed by recommended methods, and a look to the future of population control.

Produced by the Health Education Audio-Visual for the British Medical Association. Obtained from Health Education Audio-Visual, 24 Bryanston Street, London W.1.

Family Planning

This strip concentrates initially on the population explosion throughout the world, followed again by clear pictures of unreliable and reliable methods of birth control. Clear, bright simple frames. *Available from Camera Talks, 31 North Row, London W.1, on sale or return basis (see above).*

Many more films, filmstrips and books on all aspects of sexuality, from early adolescence, through marriage, parenthood and family life, are listed in the following booklets: *Resource List—Responsible Parenthood and Sex Education* and *A Selection of Films for Family Planning Programmes,* both from the International Planned Parenthood Federation, 18–20 Lower Regent Street, London SW1 4PW. *Book List 1982* from The Family Planning Association, 27–35 Mortimer Street, London W1A 4QW.

SLIDES

The following slides relate to pregnancy, labour and birth control.
Birth Atlas Slide Series
A set of 22 slides adapted from the Birth Atlas drawings shown against a coloured background. It includes male and female reproductive organs and a breech delivery. Text of accompanying booklet is available in French, Spanish and English.
Available from Maternity Center Association, 48 East 92nd Street, New York N.Y. 10028

A New Life—Cow & Gate teaching aid. 35 slides. These are identical to the Cow & Gate flip chart and are accompanied by an explanatory booklet.
Cow & Gate Baby Foods, Guildford, Surrey.

The Development of the Foetus 12 slides
These slides are sold with a teachers' booklet and are taken from the film *The first days of life.* See films.

Care During Pregnancy 12 slides
These show diet, rest, nutrition, posture, exercise and antenatal care.

Again sold with a teachers' booklet.
Last two available from the E.P. Group of Companies, Educational Products Ltd, East Ardsley, Wakefield, Yorks.

The Expectant Father 86 × 35 mm colour slides, with teaching notes, *Part 1.* Pregnancy and birth

Inevitably, this concentrates on what is going on inside the woman, and how she keeps fit during pregnancy. The father's feelings about breast and bottle feeding are touched on, and he is encouraged to stop smoking and eat healthily with his partner. The couple are filmed discussing major decisions, such as moving house, and planning the baby's equipment together. The roles of midwife and physiotherapist are shown, with an antenatal class and clinic attendance. The birth is viewed from the mother's angle.

Part 2. Afterwards

These slides are photographs interspersed with cartoons, and bring in the father's role well, as helper, supporter, ally and comforter. Some of the cartoons, such as the one of father driving away hordes of visitors with a dustbin lid and a broom, and, later, another of the father shut out while mother is surrounded by crowds of her friends and their babies, make their point clearly and humorously.

The midwife, family doctor, health visitor and health clinic are all shown, but it is stated that soon the parents will know their baby better than all the professionals. Various details such as, for instance, safe equipment, grandparents as baby-sitters, and the family planning clinic, could all be enlarged upon as each teacher wishes while using the slides.

They were produced in conjunction with Plymouth Health Authority's Health Education Service, and their aim is to 'make expectant fathers feel included in pregnancy, in an effort to build a closer bond between both parents and their child.'

For sale from Farley Health Products Ltd., Torr Lane, Plymouth, Devon.

SLIDES WITH TAPES

Birth Control Methods 20 slides, cassette, booklet describing the slides (contained in a plastic folder)

Clear slides of all recognised methods. The booklet indicates when the slides should be changed as the slides run.

From Schering Educational Services, Schering Chemicals Ltd, Burgess Hill, Sussex.

Safe Sex Contraception Kit (boxed)
Forty-eight slides with a tape. (The tape has musical intervals after each section so that it can be stopped to allow discussion.) A cue sheet is provided, indicating the material on the tape.

Also includes all recognised contraceptive products, and 20 *Safe Sex* leaflets in each kit.

Available from Birmingham Brook Advisory Centre, Educational Services, 9 York Road, Edgbaston, Birmingham.

Local Family Planning Services will often supply, on free loan, a Contraceptive Display Kit.

Having a Baby in Britain 72 slides
These are useful for all teachers who have a large immigrant Asian population as they enable the group to understand, even if non-English speaking, the important aspects of pregnancy and birth, as slides are of Asian families, and are informative and interesting.

The slides have to be bought in their entirety, but in fact are divided into five parts, to provide a nucleus of five lessons. Each part after the first, reminds the group of the previous session before continuing.

The first part deals with antenatal care, hospital booking and routine. The second—*How to look after yourself*—diet exercise, antenatal classes, posture and positive health. The third, fourth and fifth show the first stage of labour, birth and how to cope after the baby is born.

One great advantage of these slides is that Asian mothers can identify with the pictures culturally. The second is that they are supplied with relevant tapes and a book of directions in English (when to change the slide, and a description of the next one) so that a teacher can know what information is on the tape.

The tapes can be supplied in Hindi, Gujerati, Urdu, Bengali, Punjabi and English, and can be bought separately.

Obtainable from the Medical Audio-Visual Library, P.O. Box 99, Chelmsford.

FILM LOOPS

Super 8 mm colour film loop, approximately 4 minutes each
Childbirth
    Labour in animated diagrams.

The Birth of a Baby
  Childbirth in live action.
'Baby Feeding from Birth' Series
  Breast Feeding
  Preparing a Bottle Feed
  Preparing Spoonfeeds
'Babycare' Series
  Eight film loops, including bathing, nappy changing, breast and bottle feeding.
All available from Eothen Films Ltd., E.M.I. Studios, Borehamwood, Hertfordshire.

Also, short 8 mm film sequences, mounted in cassettes, showing breathing, relaxation, posture, lifting and postnatal exercises are available from Camera Talks.

POSTERS

There are many extremely bright posters available, but few portray immigrants. However, there is a very good poster available from the Health Education Council, of a most attractive Indian girl, breast feeding, which could encourage others to do likewise.

USEFUL ADDRESSES

A teacher should try to collect a 'portfolio' of useful addresses from which added information and help can be obtained by members of her class. Here are a few that we have found useful.

The Borough or County Health Education Officer. Contact can be made through the District Health Department, Personal Health Section.

Local health visitors and midwives and their methods of working (are they area-based or attached to general practitioner teams? The latter is becoming much more common now, so that a teacher, on knowing the name of a class member's GP, can say, 'Your health visitor is . . . and can be contacted at . . .').

Local hospitals, how to get there, and the procedure each requires to inform them when the mother is in labour.

Local ambulance station phone numbers, and which to telephone when in labour. (Information has to be kept up to date. One of us has recently had to tell classes that the ambulance number has changed, and from now on women in labour should dial 999.)

The local Health and Social Security Department.

The local Social Services Department. This department now, as well as its many other activities, organises the Home Help Service.

The Health Visitors Association—the professional body for all health visitors, 36 Eccleston Square, London S.W. 1. Tel. 01-834 9523.

The Royal College of Midwives—the professional body for midwives, 15 Mansfield Street, London W.1. Tel. 01-580 6523.

The Association of Chartered Physiotherapists in Obstetrics and Gynaecology can be contacted through the professional body for physiotherapists—The Chartered Society of Physiotherapy at 14 Bedford Row, London W.C.1. Telephone 01-242 1941. Regional representatives of this body will have details of hospital classes in their area. Members also run courses, hold a stock of books and publish a newsletter.

The Health Education Council has lists of useful addresses and publishes free leaflets and posters in different languages on many aspects of health education including preparation for pregnancy and labour. 78 New Oxford Street, London W.C.1. Telephone 01-637 1881.

The National Childbirth Trust headquarters, 9 Queensborough Terrace, London W.2. Telephone 01-229 9319. Since the 1950s the Trust, of which both authors are life members, has encouraged the establishment and maintenance of good antenatal classes and attempted to achieve conditions to make childbearing as satisfying an experience as possible for all women. More recently they have sponsored postnatal support groups and breast feeding promotion groups all over the country. Lists of Trust leaflets, books and aids can be obtained from N.C.T. (Maternity Sales Ltd), 9 Queensborough Terrace, London W2 3TB. Addresses of teachers, organisers and counsellors can be obtained from headquarters.

The Birth Centre is a meeting place for people who are concerned about the increasing mechanisation of birth and who favour birth in an atmosphere of love and care with full participation of both parents. Information about activities, including film and discussion evenings, from Mrs Claxton, 16 Simpson Street, London SW11.

A.I.M.S. A pressure group for better care of women in pregnancy and labour and the happiness and well-being of all mothers. c/o Christine Beels, 19 Broomfield Crescent, Leeds 6. Telephone Leeds (0532) 751911.

La Leche League. An international association started in the U.S.A. to promote breast feeding. English representative at P.O. Box BM2434, London WC1 6XX.

Foresight. An organisation dedicated to good pre-conceptual care. Publishes handbooks, holds meetings and organises a growing number of clinics where couples can go for check-ups. Woodhurst, Hydestile, Godalming, Surrey.

Association of Radical Midwives. This association was founded in 1976, to encourage midwives in their support of a woman's active participation in labour, and also to re-establish the confidence of the midwife in her own skills. They are trying to be truly, as their name, 'with the woman', in labour, and throughout the parturition period. c/o Sally Hart, Haringey Women's Centre, 40 Turnpike Lane, London N4. Telephone 01 889 3912.

Active Birth Movement. A new association dedicated to the exponents of activity in labour and freedom for women to choose their own position for delivery. Runs conferences, lectures and classes. Janet Balaskas, 32 Cholmeley Crescent, Highgate, London N6. Telephone 01 348 1284.

Imprints. Birth and Life Bookstore produce a review, newsletter catalogue of mainly but not entirely American books, leaflets and films on childbirth and childrearing. Subscribers recieve the newsletter twice a year and can order books on the form provided and pay by international money order. Delivery is very rapid.

The nearest Family Planning Centre, with times of opening, appointment systems, and how to make the appointment. This information can be obtained from local clinics or health centres.

The National Council for One-Parent Families, 255 Kentish Town Road, London N.W.5. Telephone 01-267 1361. (Each local authority has a social welfare section to help unmarried mothers, sometimes called 'Welcare'. Information on the whereabouts of this section can be obtained from the above or from local Social Service Departments).

Gingerbread. (An organisation to help unsupported parents and their children—run by volunteers, who hold group meetings, discuss and help with problems and try to find accommodation.) Information from their headquarters, Gingerbread, 9 Poland Street, London W.1. Telephone 01-734 9014.

Local mothers' clubs and groups. These may be held in church halls, but very many are in clinics and health centres. The mothers have talks, demonstrations, bring-and-buy sales, sometimes keep-fit classes, while the babies and toddlers are cared for by others—in clinics these are trained nurses or nursery nurses, with volunteer mothers. These clubs can be a valuable social outlet to a new mother and often the members can be extremely supportive to each other.

The nearest marriage guidance councillors (obtainable from the Headquarters, Marriage Guidance Council, 76A New Cavendish Street, London W.1. Telephone 01-580 1087.)

Relaxation for Living. Started by a National Childbirth Trust member, and now country-wide. Groups are taught how to erase tension from everyday life, and deep relaxation is taught by different methods. More information from the group's founder, Mrs Amber Lloyd, Dunesk, 29 Burwood Park Road, Walton-on-Thames. Telephone Walton 27826.

International Childbirth Education Association. This group, based in the U.S.A., issues a useful news-sheet on preparation for child-birth and allied subjects, reviews new teaching material in English and provides a supply centre from which books published in America and Canada can easily be obtained. Payment is arranged through a bank or by international money order. ICEA Supplies Center, P.O. Box 70258, Seattle, Washington 98107.

Some resource centres, books, films, and teaching aids from overseas

We are very grateful to our overseas contributors, who have supplied all the following information.

AMERICA

Compiled by Jayne Wiggins

Books

This list suggests a few of the books in the several categories relating to childbearing and childrearing. It is just a sampling.

Beals, P. (1980) *Parent's Guide to the Childbearing Year*.
Source book for expectant parents.

Bing, E. & Coleman, L. (1977) *Making Love during Pregnancy*.
Practical guide to dispel myths about having intercourse during pregnancy.

Bonica, J. (1980) *Obstetrical Analgesia and Anesthesia*.
Classic work on pain relief for childbirth, organised in logical sequence, written for professionals.

Boston Women's Health Club Collective (1979) *Our bodies, Ourselves: a Book by and for Women.*
Comprehensive 'course' on biological and physiological functioning of women.

Bradley, R. (1981) 3rd edn. *Husband-coached Childbirth.*
How a husband can help his wife during pregnancy and childbirth.

Dick-Read, G. (1972) 4th ed. *Childbirth without Fear.*
Incorporates the best of Dick-Read's writings, principles, practice and biography.

Dolane, J (1976) *Group Organisation Guide.*
Comprehensive guide to formation and administration of a childbirth education group.

Edwards, M. (1978) *Teenage Parents.*
Issues related to early childbearing, service programs for young expectant parents.

Donovan, B. (1978) *The Caesarean Birth Experience.*
Practical, comprehensive and reassuring guide for parents and professionals.

Eiger, J. & Olds, S. (1972) *The Complete Book of Breastfeeding.*
Comprehensive, easy reading. Good discussion of sexual aspects.

Feldman, S. (1978) *Choices in Childbirth.*
Discussion of alternatives in childbirth, from technological-aided hospital birth to midwife attended home birth.

Fraiberg, S. (1959) *The Magic Years.*
Offers insight into interior life of infant and young child.

Haire, D. (Pamphlet) *Instructions for Nursing your Baby.*
Also available in French and Spanish.

Kitzinger, S. (1978) *The Experience of Childbirth,* 4th edn.
Introduction to childbirth; focusses on psychological aspects of childbearing.

Klaus, M. & Kennel, J. (1981) *Parent-infant Bonding.* 2nd edn.
Discusses experiences of individual family members during pregnancy, childbirth and care of siblings.

LaLeche League, International *The Womanly Art of Breastfeeding.*
Practical manual for instruction and support to nursing mothers.

Lamaze, F. (1965) *Painless Childbirth.*
Classic book to giving birth the natural way.

National Association of Childbirth Education (1980) *El Cuidado Prenatal y Preparacion para el Parto: Quia Completa*.
Supplement for Spanish-speaking persons attending Lamaze classes.

Nilsson, L., et. al. (1977) *A Child is Born*.
Human reproduction from conception to birth. Outstanding photographs.

Noble, E. (1980) *Having Twins, a Parent's Guide to Pregnancy, Childbirth and Early Parenthood*.
Prenatal care, parenting tips and facts dealing with multiple births.

Oxorn, H. (1980) 4th. ed. *Human Labor and Birth*.
Basic textbook on normal obstretrics.

Phillips, C. & Anzalone, J. (1978) *Fathering*.
Supplemental text for professionals on active father participation in childbirth.

Pryor, L. (1973) *Nursing your Baby*.
Informative discussion of how the breasts function, and week-by-week guide.

Ribble, M. (1965) *The Rights of Infants*, 2nd edn.
Classic on basic needs of babies and the vital part mothering plays in normal development of children.

Shanteau, D. (1981) *Audio Visuals about Birth and Family Life*.
Descriptive listing of over 800 audio-visuals with distributor, rental and purchase information.

Wiggins, J. (1979) *Childbearing: Physiology, Experiences, Needs*.
Readable reference on normal obstetrics designed for expectant parents and childbirth educators.

Worthington, B. et. al. (1981) *Nutrition in Pregnancy and Lactation*. 2nd edn.
All aspects of maternal nutrition are discussed.

Guidance

Local and state departments of health offer guidance in setting up or improving family centered maternity services, and on safety standards. In addition, help may be obtained from:

U.S. Consumer Product Safety Commission
Washington, D.C., 2027
Toll free phone 800-492-2937
Provides information on safety standards for cribs, toys and other accessories for children. Many booklets also available.

U.S. Government
Health and Human Services
Hyattsville, Maryland 20780
> A government agency concerned with health and welfare of the population.

Journals

An increasing number of professional and/or lay magazines are devoted to the broad topic of perinatology. The most widely known are:

Journal of Nurse-Midwifery
Suite 1120
1522 K Street N.W.
Washington, D.C.
> The official journal of the American College of Nurse-Midwifery.

Journal of Obstetrics, Gynecologic and Neonatal
Nursing (JOGN)
Lippincott/Harper, Publishers
Subscribers Services Department
P.O. Box 1600
Hagerstown, Maryland 21740
> The professional journal of NAACOG.

Birth and the Family Journal (BFJ)
110 El Camino Real
Berkeley, California 94705
> For the serious childbirth educator and parent advocate.

Briefs
Maternity Center Association
48 E. 92 Street
New York, New York 10028
> Digest magazine covering latest developments in maternity and child care.

ICEA News
(See ICEA address under Organisations)
Official publication of ICEA

The American Journal of Maternal Child Nursing (MCN)
555 West 57 Street
New York, New York 10019
> Designed for use by nurses interested in maternal child nursing.

Organisations

Numerous national/international organisations are dedicated to improving standards of care, assisting and supporting safe birth alternatives and providing educational materials for expectant and new parents.

Many of these organisations have local or regional chapters. For specifics contact the parent organisation. It is the best means of getting up-to-date information.

Pertinent continuing education programmes and regional conferences are offered by these organisations. Information about these and about teacher-training programmes can be obtained by contacting the national headquarters.

Guidelines, statements, technical bulletins and documents relating to perinatal care are periodically published, particularly by NAACOG, the Cooperative Birth Center and the American College of Nurse-Midwifery.

American Academy of Husband-coached Childbirth
P.O. Box 5224
Sherman Oaks, California 91413
Teaches Robert Bradley's method of husband-coached childbirth, an offshoot of Grantly Dick-Read method.

American Academy of Pediatrics
P.O. Box 1034
Evanston, Illinois 60204
Provides literature for parents and professionals relating to child care, illness and welfare.

American National Red Cross
17 and D Streets
Washington, D.C. 20006
Sponsors classes for expectant parents throughout the country.

American Physical Therapy Association
OB/GYN Section
1156 15th Street N.W.
Washington, D.C. 20005
Promotes active involvement of physical therapists in the Ob/Gyn area.

American Society of Childbirth Educators
19 D-230 Riverside Drive
New York, New York 10025
An organisation of childbirth educators with backgrounds of nursing/nurse midwifery and education, dedicated to the maintenance of high standards in the field of parent education.

American Society for Psychoprophylaxis in Obstetrics (ASPO)
1523 L. Street N.W.
Washington, D.C. 20005
Emphasises Lamaze technique of preparation for childbirth.

Caesarean/Support, Education and Concern (C/SEC)
15 Maynard Road

Dedham, Massachusetts 02026
Chapters throughout the country offer emotional and physical support to
parents who have had Caesarean births.

Child Study Association (CSA)
853 Broadway
New York, New York 10028
Provides educational materials for parents.

Cooperative Birth Centre Network
Box 1 Route 1
Perklomenville, Pennsylvania 18074
'To assist and support the development and accessibility of safe, cost
efficient birth alternatives, with particular attention to the out-of-hospital
birth center.'

International Childbirth Education Association (ICEA)
Box 20048
Minneapolis, Minnesota 55420
An interdisciplinary organisation representing groups and individuals
sharing an interest in family centered maternity care.

LaLeche League International
9616 Minneapolis Avenue
Franklin Park, Illinois 60131
Chapters throughout the world, sponsoring, encouraging and teaching
breast feeding.

Maternity Center Association (MCA)
48 East 92 Street
New York, New York 10028
An internationally known health organisation dedicated to meeting the
needs of parents by conducting classes for them, workshops to prepare
professionals to teach, developing and distributing teaching aids and
publishing Briefs.

National Association of Parents and Professionals
for Safe Alternatives in Childbirth (NAPSAC)
P.O. Box 267
Marble Hill, Missouri 63764
Seeks to provide safe alternatives to traditional childbirth methods
throughout the United States.

National Foundation/March of Dimes
1275 Mamaroneck Avenue
White Plains, New York 10605
Aims to improve level of care of all people with birth defects. Sponsors
workshops, has available publications pertinent to defects.

National Organisation of Twins Club
5402 Amberwood Lane
Rockville, Maryland 20853
Chapters throughout the United States, providing opportunity to share problems of other mothers of twins.

Parents Without Partners
7901 Woodmont Avenue
Bethesda, Maryland 20014
Aimed at guiding parents without partners, and their children, in coping with their special problems.

Planned Parenthood Federation of America
501 Madison Avenue
New York, New York 10022
Provides leadership for universal acceptance of family planning as an element of responsible family life.

Sex Information and Educational Council of the
United States (SIECUS)
80 Fifth Avenue Suite 801
New York, New York 10011
National clearing house for information on human sexuality. Six times a year publishes SEICUS Report and Bibliographies. Resources and library open to students and professionals.

The Nurses Association of the American College of
Obstetricians and Gynecologists (NAACOG)
600 Maryland Avenue S. W. Suite 200
Washington, D.C. 20024
This professional organisation promotes the highest standards of obstetric, gynecologic and neonatal nursing practice, cooperating at all levels with qualified physicians and nurses; and stimulating interest in obstetric, gynecologic and neonatal nursing.

Resource centers

Some organisations* offering guidelines, teacher-training workshops, professional statements of purpose, information about continuing education, general information and bibliographies are:

American Society for Psychoprophylaxis in Obstetrics (ASPO)

Cooperative Birth Center Network

International Childbirth Education Association (ICEA)

Maternity Center Association

* For address see Organisation

National Foundation/March of Dimes

The Nursing Association of the American College of Obstetricians and Gynecologists (NAACOG)

Sources of films, bibliographies, books

Some parent/professional groups publish newsletters, reviews of new materials and maintain supply centres from which materials can be ordered directly.

The ICEA has available the following:

* Bookmarks—reviews of new books and short descriptions of all books and pamphlets available from ICEA Book Centers.
* Review—published several times yearly, each issue focussed on one subject of current interest. Abstracts are included.
* Film Directory—lists current films and other visual aids, and their sources.

It is sometimes possible to borrow or rent films from local libraries, local and state health departments and film libraries, and parent education groups, as well as from the film distributors.

The latest information about books on childbearing and related subjects may be obtained from publishing companies known for their books on the subjects.

Consumer Information Center
(United States Government Printing Office)
Pueblo, Colorado 81009

Health Services Administration
Executive Secretariat
5600 Fischer Lane
Rockville, Maryland 20857
Extensive listing of publications and teaching aids in Spanish.

Imprints
Birth and Life Bookstore
Review Newsletter and Catalog
P. O. Box 70625
Seattle, Washington 98107

* International Childbirth Education Association (ICEA)

* Maternity Center Association (MCA)

Naissance-Renaissance
891 des Erables CP 2363
St. Nicholas—Est
Quebec GOS 3 LO
Canada
Information concerning publications in French

*For addresses see Organisations

J. B. Lippincott Company
Health Professionals Publications
East Washington Square
Philadelphia, Pennsylvania 19106

Little, Brown and Company
34 Beacon Street
Boston, Massachusetts 02106

McGraw-Hill Book Company
P.O. Box 400
Hightstown, New Jersey 08520

The C. V. Mosby Company
11830 Westline Industrial Drive
St. Louis, Missouri 63141

W. B. Saunders
West Washington Square
Philadelphia, Pennsylvania 19105

Teaching aids

The sources of teaching aids range from organisations to commercial
companies. These companies offer such items as pamphlets, films, and
samples of products.

Abbott Laboratories
North Chicago, Illinois 60064

Ayerst Laboratories
685 Third Avenue
New York, New York 10017

Carnation
Medical Marketing
5405 Wilshire
Los Angeles, California 90036

Childbirth Educational Supply Center
10 Sol Drive
Carmel, New York 10512

Corometrics Medical Systems, Inc.
Director of Medical Education
Box 333, 61 Barnes Park Road North
Wallingford, Connecticut 06492

Evenflow Products Company
771 North Freedom Street
Ravenna, Ohio 44266

Lifecircle
2378-Cornell Drive
Cosa Mesa, California 92926

Johnson and Johnson
Products Director
Grandview Road
Skillman, New Jersey 08558

Gerber Products Company
Medical Marketing Services
445 State Street
Freemont, Michigan 49412

Lederle Laboratories
Pearl River, New York 10965

Mead Johnson and Company
Evansville, Indiana 47721

Mennan Company
Professional Service Department
Morristown, New Jersey 07960

Ortho Corporation
Raritan, New Jersey 08869

Pfizer, Incorporated
Leeming Division
100 Jefferson Road
Parsippany, New Jersey 07054

Proctor and Gamble Company
Professional Service Division
Box 171
Cincinnati, Ohio 45201

Ross Laboratories
Department of Nursing Service
Columbus, Ohio 43216

Shering Corporation
Galloping Hill Road
Kenilworth, New Jersey 07033

Wyeth Laboratories
Philadelphia, Pennsylvania 19101

Films

The following is just a sampling of the many films, slides, cassettes and video-cassettes which have been produced by individuals and groups, including professional, lay and commercial organisations. They may be previewed, rented or purchased directly from the sources indicated.

Some parents' organisations, professional organisations, libraries and universities have rental services.

For information about Braille teaching aids and audio-aids, write to:

Library of Congress
Reference section
Division for blind and physically handicapped
Washington, D.C. 20542

A comprehensive directory may be purchased from ICEA: Caldwell, L. (ed.) (1978) *ICEA Film Directory with Teaching Aids Supplement*

Dar Pecho (Spanish) Film

Preparation for breast feeding.
Videograph
2833 25th Street
San Francisco, California 94110

The Caesarean experience Film

Indications for Caesarean section, and vaginal delivery after Caesarean section.
Artemis
19460 Stratford
Detroit, Michigan 48221

Family choices: hospital options 80 color slides

Three births show vaginal birth of twins, father participation and sibling participation.
Artemis
19460 Stratford
Detroit, Michigan 48221

Fathers: a film portrait Film

Focusses on the father in the context of the childbearing period.
ASPO
1411 K Street NW
Washington, D.C. 20005

Five women, five births Films, slides, cassette, video-cassette

Emotional aspects and views of five births: 2 at home, a breech hospital birth, a Caesarean birth and a hospital delivery of a prepared mother.

Artemis
19460 Stratford
Detroit, Michigan 48221

Maternidad (Spanish) Film

Preparation for childbearing.
Childbirth Education Films
Videograph
2833 25th Street
San Francisco, California 94110

Midwife Film

Discussion of midwifery practice; shows two home births.
Cinema Media
664 North Michigan Avenue
Chicago, Illinois 60611

Midwife: with woman Film

The history of midwifery, and births at a free-standing birth center.
Maternity Center Association
48 East 92 Street
New York, N.Y. 10025

Nicholas and the baby Film, video-cassette,

Sibling's reaction to the coming of a new baby.
Center Productions Inc.
1327 Spruce Street #3
Boulder, Colorado 80302

Nutrition in pregnancy Film

Emphasises critical importance of nutrition during pregnancy.
Jay Hathaway Productions
4846 Katherine Avenue
Sherman Oaks, California 91423

Preparation for breastfeeding Slides, cassette

Shows physical methods of preparing the breasts for breast feeding.
Educational Graphics Aids
1315 Norwood
Boulder, Colorado 80302

Squatting birth film. Film

Shows mother delivering baby while squatting.
CMI
2335 West Foster Avenue
Chicago, Illinois 60625

AUSTRALIA

Compiled by D. Jones and E. Burman

State secretaries of obstetric physiotherapy groups

Australian Capital Territory

Mrs Joyce Luck
15 Weingarth Street
Holder, A.C.T. 2611

New South Wales

Mrs Jill Marshall
1 Fernleigh Road
Caringbah, NSW 2229

Queensland

Mrs Lorrie Ormiston
35 Scherger Street
Moonooka, Q. land. 4105

South Australia

Mrs Pam Lane
P.O. Box 444
Gawler, S.A. 5118

Tasmania

Mrs Helen Lawrence
165 Davey Street
Hobart, Tas. 7000

Victoria

Mrs Barbara Reid
21 Dean Street
Kew, Vic. 3101

Western Australia

Mrs Kaye Brand
10 Hawk Grove
Burrendah. W.A. 6155

Northern Territory

Mrs Jennifer Woodhouse
4 Crush Street
Fannie Bay, N.T. 5790

Resource centres

The Australian Physiotherapy Association
234 Albert Road
South Melbourne
Victoria 3205
03 690 5533

Nursing Mothers' Association of Australia National Headquarters
357 Burwood Road
Hawthorn
Victoria 3122
03 818 8031

Parent Centres
83 Albert Drive
Killara 2071

Childbirth & Parenting Association
13 Hull Road
Croydon
Victoria 3136

Childbirth Education Association (Aust.)
116 Glenferrie Road
Malvern 3144
Victoria
03 509 9985

Family Planning Association
270 Church Street
Richmond 3121
Victoria
03 428 1414

There are branches of the above Associations in most States so please consult
your State's telephone directory.

Books

Auckett, A. D. (1981) *Baby Massage*. Melbourne: Hill of Content
Beischer, N. & Mackay, E. (1976) *Obstetrics and the Newborn*. Sydney: Holt-Saunders.
Brook, D. (1977) *Naturebirth*. Melbourne: Penguin.
Gold, S. & Eisen, P. (1969) *How to Bring up Your Parents*. Melbourne: Sun Books.
Isbister, C. (1963) *Preparing for Motherhood*. Sydney: Angus & Robertson.
Isbister, C. (1971) *Birth, Infancy and Childhood*, 2nd edn. Sydney: Farleigh Press.
Isbister, C. (1976) *Birth of a Family*. Melbourne: Nelson.
Leeton, J. (1974) *All about Birth Control*. Sydney: Nelson.
Lennane, J. & Lennane, J. (1977) *Hard Labour—Realists' Guide to Having a Baby*. Melbourne: Hutchinson.
Llewellyn Jones, D. (1969) *Fundamentals of Obstetrics and Gynaecology*, Vol. 1. London: Faber & Faber.
Llewellyn Jones, D. (1974) *Human Reproduction and Society*. London: Faber & Faber.
Llewellyn Jones, D. (1978) *Everywoman*, 2nd edn. London: Faber & Faber.
Lumley, J. & Astbury, J. (1980) *Birth rites, Birth rights or Childbirth Alternatives for Australian Parents*. Melbourne: Sphere Books.
Mayle, P. (1977) *How to be a Pregnant Father*. Melbourne: Sun Books.
Meares, A. (1967) *Relief without Drugs*. Glasgow: Collins.
O'Brien, P. (1979) *Discovering Childbirth and the Joy of Breastfeeding*. Sydney: Angus & Robertson.
Phillips, V. (1976) *Successful Breastfeeding*. Melbourne: Hedges & Bell.
Townsend, L. (1969) *Obstetrics for Students*, 2nd edn. Melbourne: Melbourne University Press.
Wood, C. & Reed, D. (1973) *ABZ of Pregnancy*. Melbourne: Dominion Press.

Booklets

Childbirth Education Association (1977) *A Gentle Welcome*. Melbourne: Action Printing.
Childbirth Education Association (N.S.W.) (1979) *A Guide to Labour*. Contributed by Brittlebank, Dip. Phys. M.A.P.A., Browne, B.Sc. (Phys.) M.A.P.A. Booker, D.S.C.M. (P & T).
Childbirth and Parenting Association of Victoria Ltd., Caesar Support Group, P.O. Box 480, Ringwood 3134. *What about Birth by Caesarean Section?*
Clare, A. & Thomas, M. (1973) *All about Childbirth*. Australia: Rigby.
Karitaine Mothercraft Society (1974) *An Approach to Fatherhood*. Sydney.
Mother and Babies' Health Association. *Preparing for Childbirth*. Adelaide.
Obstetric Physiotherapy Society of Victoria. *Physiotherapy Advice for New Mothers—Take care of yourself as well as your baby—Back Care*.
Prepare for Your Birth Day —Publicity Brochure.

Physiotherapy—Prenatal body care and exercise—Exercise Sheet.
Nutrition in Pregnancy—Reprint from Australian Baby Talk.
Available from Obstetric Physiotherapy Society of Victoria, c/o Australian
Physiotherapy Association Headquarters, 302A Queens Parade, Clifton
Hill, Victoria.
Booklets on Breastfeeding, Crying, Cot Death, etc. are available from
Nursing Mothers Association, Australia, and Parents Centres, Australia.

Tapes

Gibson, M. & Ritchie, R. *Prepared Childbirth*. Childbirth Education
Association.
Vines, L. & Chung, I. *Nerves*. Australian College of Recorded Education,
Olivetti House, 140 Williams Street, Sydney 2000.
Vines, L. *Stress Management in Early Parenthood*. Australian College of
Recorded Education, Olivetti House, 140 Williams Street, Sydney 2000.
Hickey, J. *Childbirth—tape for class teaching*. Parents Centres Australia,
P.O. Box 234, Glebe, N.S.W. 2037.
Walker, B. *Labour Rehearsal* (to be produced 1983). Obstetric Physio-
therapy Society of Victoria.
The Obstetric Physiotherapy Groups of New South Wales and Victoria run
a cassette library from which many tapes can be borrowed. Address through
Obstetric Physiotherapy Group of New South Wales and Victoria.

Films

For the love of a child Produced by Childbirth Education Association,
Victoria, 50 minutes.
Home Birth Baby. Leboyer-home delivery, 8 minutes.
Breastfeeding—What a Beautiful Thing to Do. Nursing Mothers Association
of Australia, 35 minutes.
Breastfeeding. Nursing Mothers Association, Victorian Branch, c/o 11 St
Agnes Court, Avondale Heights 3034, 15 minutes.
For Better for Worse (1979) Family Planning Association Tasmania, 20
minutes.
Birth & Beyond. Homebirth, Nimbin, N.S.W. 25 minutes.
Harmony in Pregnancy, Harmony at Birth, Harmony Parents Centres, N.S.W.
Emotional Aspects of Pregnancy. Educational Media, Melbourne.
Don't Cry Baby. Produced by Childbirth Education Association, Sydney.
Available Childbirth Education Association, Sydney and Melbourne,
black and white, 10 minutes.
You are Only Born Once. Produced by Doug Stomley for Childbirth
Education Association, from 116 Glenferrie Road, Malvern 3144, 30
minutes.
A Gentle Birth. Australian Film and Television School, 13 Lyon Park Road,
North Ryde, N.S.W. 2113.
Birth to Walking. Film Australia, Elton Road, Lindfield, N.S.W. 2070.

CANADA

Compiled by Iris Weverman

Films by company

Modern Talking Picture Service—areas across Canada

Central Branch:
143 Sparks Avenue
Willowdale, Ontario
M2H 2S5

Your New Baby, 11.23 minutes care of newborn. Free rental
A Good Start, 13.09 minutes infant feeding
Baby Feeding and Nutrition, 24 minutes breast feeding and nutrition

Procter and Gamble Inc.

c/o Professional Services Division
P.O. Box 355, Station A
Toronto, Ontario
M5W IC5

First Two Weeks of Life
Parenting Experience
Your New Baby and You

Omega Films

133 Manville Road, Unit 19
Scarborough, Ontario
M1C 4J7
Telephone No. 416-755-1140

Baby Dance
15 minutes
Film about pregnancy and fitness.

First steps
12 minutes
Animated film about pregnancy, childbirth, infant development and parenting.

Wyeth Limited Library

4455 Chesswood Drive—free loan
Toronto, Ontario.
Telephone No. 630-0280

Beginning of Life 30 minutes
Colour photography shows fertilisation of an ovum and the course it takes from there.

Breast Feeding 10 minutes

Infant Feeding some nutritional considerations, 27 minutes

Films

Ross Audiovisual Library

4980 rue Buchan
Montreal, Quebec, Canada.
H4P IS9
Telephone No. 514-735-2246
Ontario Branch 416-499-1400
British Columbia 604-738-3161
Free loaning library—films available for purchase

Code:
9185 *Breast Feeding : The Natural Way*, 15 minutes English/French
8183 *Formula Preparation*, 25 minutes, English *newborn* 1 to 7 days
9016 *Amazing Newborn*, 25 minutes, English explored
9040 *Death of a Newborn*, 32 minutes, English, Dr Marshall Klaus

National Film Board—offices across Canada

Central branch:
1 Lombard Street
Toronto, Ontario
M5C 1J6
Telephone No. English 369-4092
French 369-4110
Free loan—pay postage
Newborn Birthright 28 minutes
Postpartum Depression 28 minutes, excellent, A self help group discussing postpartum issues.

Kinetic Film Enterprises—write for catalogue for movie films

781 Gerrard Street East
Toronto, Ontario
M4M 1Y5
Telephone No. 416-469-4155
Nan's Class 40 minutes, six different births, family care and role of the coach.
A Labour of Love 31 minutes, a family centered childbirth with father and sibling participation.
Caesarean Childbirth 16 minutes, what is c/s? Why do you have . . . etc.
Pregnancy after 35 14 minutes

It's Not an Illness 23 minutes a film on fitness and pregnancy
Breastfeeding—a special closeness 23 minutes

City Films

542 Gordon Baker Road
Willowdale Ont. M2H 3B4
Telephone 416-499-1400
All films are available to be purchased.
Bonding Birth Experience 21 minutes
The emphasis on the motions of labour and birth.
Breast Feeding Experience 24 minutes
This film has a hospital with a baby who has trouble breastfeeding.
Pregnant Fathers 28 minutes
A sensitive film of a prepared childbirth concentrating on the father's role.
Shared Beginning 26 minutes
Shared Caesarean Section 28 minutes
The Canadian film of a couple's first child by Caesarean section.
Family Birthing
Multipurpose film showing low risk childbirth, births in hospital in a birth centre, care by nurse midwives, family centred care, family infant bonding, three births.
Born Drunk. The Fetal Alcohol Syndrome, 10 minutes
The Superbaby. Parenting Kit.
Filmstrip with cassette, wall charts, activity sheets, teacher's guide, additional audio cassette *Pregnant Moments*. Devised by numerous consultants in the Toronto Area.

Slides

Pregnancy
You and Your Baby slide/cassette presentation, 14 minutes, 35 mm, colour slide, Available from Ross Laboratories, Division of Abbot Laboratories Limited, Montreal, Canada, H4P 1A5
Price: free to keep

Slide presentation

Dental presentation   Ontario Dental Association
26 minutes—slide and tape   234 St. George Street
discussion on fluoride; baby   Toronto, Ontario.
teeth etc.

Tapes

Relaxation in Daily Living and as a Therapeutic Technique
PHY # 5
Dorothy Clarke Madgett

Available from:
Audio Archives of Canada
7449 Victoria Park
Markham, Ontario
L3R 2Y7

Relaxation Programme
30 minutes
Dr L. J. Goldsmith
Canadian Back Education Unit
Burton Hall
60 Grosvenor Street
Toronto, Ontario

Magazine

Great Expectation
Professional Publishing Associates
30 Bloor Street West
Toronto, Ontario
M4N 1A2
4 × year
Free to new parents in classes

American journals

Excellent!
Birth and the Family Journal
published quarterly by ICEA & ASPO
110 El Camino Real
Berkeley California
U.S.A. 94705

American Baby Magazine
published monthly
352 Evelyn Street 12/7.95
Paramus N.J. 07652
U.S.A.

Pamphlets

1. *Your Back and How to Care For It*
Schering Corp. Ltd.,
3535 Trans Canada Highway
Point Claire, Quebec
H9R 1B4

2. *Fetal Monitoring Booklet*
Hewlitt Packord

6877 Goreway Drive
Malton, Ontario Tel. 678-9430

3. *Rh Factor*—Canadian Red Cross (in your area)

4. *Breast Feeding Kit*
National Health and Welfare
Nutritional Education Unit
Ottawa, Canada
K1A 1B4

5. *Pregnancy and Diabetes*
Canadian Diabetic Association
123 Edward Street, Suite 601
Toronto, Ontario
M5G 1E2
by Juke Davis, R. P. Dt. 36 pages

6. *Premature Infant*
A handbook for parents
by Nancy Shusenberg R.N. B.Sc.N./80
Hospital for Sick Children
Rm. 1218
555 University Avenue,
Toronto, Ontario
M5G 1X8

Handout pamphlet

1. *Good Nutrition*
The Best Start In Life
Ross Laboratories
Division of Abbott Laboratories Limited
Montreal, Quebec
H4P 1A5

2. *Caesarean Birth*—A Special Delivery
5 page pamphlet
Available from Penny Press
                1100 23rd Ave. E.,
                Seattle, Washington
                98112

3. *Family Planning Resource Centre*—Free
Health & Welfare Canada
Tunney's Pasture
Oshawa, Ontario
K1A 1B5

Stock No.
6400 Can I Take This? drugs, medication during pregnancy
6466 Sex during pregnancy
6470 Sex after pregnancy

4. *Pamphlet Catalogue—Order From*
Health Information Centre
Health Promotion & Information Branch
Ministry of Health
9th Floor, Hepburn Block
Queen's Park
Toronto, Ontario
M7A 1S2
e.g. should you smoke during pregnancy?
newborn screen
nutrition
stress

5. *H. J. Heinz Company of Canada*
250 Bloor Street East
Toronto, Ontario
M4W 1E6
416-964-7057
4 pamphlets available on infant nutrition.

Pamphlets

Breast feeding Material
Available from LaLeche League (sec. resource centre)

Parenting—write for catalogue
Consumer and Corporate Affairs Canada
Consumer Services Branch
480 University Avenue, 9th Floor
Toronto, Ontario
M5G 1V2

Consumer Relations—write for material Tel, 416-924-4661
Procter and Gamble Co.—Canada Ltd.
P.O.Box 355 Station A
Toronto, Ontario
M5W 1C5 e.g. Parenting Experience

The Ontario Milk Marketing Board
Nutrition Communications
50 Maitland Avenue Tel. 416-920-2700
How to Build a Better Baby

Common Sense Parental Care—72 pages
Professional Publishing Assoc
45 Charles Street East. (LM)
Toronto, Ontario
M4Y 1S2

Gerber Foods Canada
4174 Dundas St. W., Tel. 233-2147
Toronto, Ontario.

Companies who give free information handbooks
Prudential Insurance Company
4 King Street West
Toronto, Ontario
M5H 1B7

Royal Insurance
40 Scott Street
Toronto, Ontario
M5E 1L5

Catalogues—write for each one separately

1. *P.E.R.C.* Perinatal Education Resources Communications (Free)
2820 Westminster Highway
Richmond, B.C,
V6V 1B7
604: 522-5373

2. *Life Catalogue—Life Cycle Books* (free)
2205 Danforth Avenue
Toronto, Ontario
M4C 1K4 416-690-5860— contains books, pamphlets, slides, cassettes on
pregnancy and prenatal counselling.

3. *Birth Books*—a resource for growing families
P.O. Box 836
Peterborough, Ontario
K9J 7A2
— contains audiovisual aids, pattern for knitted uterus, books, periodicals,
Schuchardt Charts, wall charts, on exercise and shape & structure of
breasts, cassettes, tapes, articles for children, e.g. cuddle carriers, and
slides.

American
4. *Childbirth Graphics*
P.O. Box 17025
Irondequoit Div. C
Rochester, New York
14617
— posters, slides, MCA Schuchardt color slides, exercise charts, handbooks, birthing models.

American
5. *Baby Dance Institute* (Owner—Elysa Markowitz)
4110 Duquesne Ave.
Culver City, Calif.
90230
— films, slides, the book 'Baby Dance', pamphlets, poster, tapes
— fitness inclined

American
6. **B.A.B.E.'S*

Bay Area Birth Education series
c/o Deanna Sollid
59 Berens Dr.
Kentfield, Ca.
94904
ph. 415-456-9181
— exercise tape and poster on pre and postnatal exercise
— slides on the Birth Experience, Hospital tour and fetal monitoring

7. *Patient Information Library*
Published by Physicians Art Service Inc.
345-G Serramonte Plaza
Poly City, CA
94105
ph. 415-994-1150
— posters and manuals of childbirth and back education and other topics
for the lay person
— 22″ × 40″ posters

Audiovisual aids

Canadian Anatomical Supply Services
308 Harbord Street
Toronto, Ontario
Canada
— bony pelvis
— bony fetal skull
— skeleton

Life Before Birth—by Lennart Nilsson
— 20 pages
— from Life Cycle Catalogue (see)
— Life Magazine Report
— excellent photography

Obstetrical Division of the Canadian Physiotherapy Association
25 Imperial Street
Toronto, Ontario
M5P 1B9
1. Prenatal wall chart—19″ × 24″
(i) large silhouettes
(ii) written exercise sheets
2. Prenatal Outline
   A guide available in English for planning prenatal classes.
3. Postnatal Outline
4. Pre and Postnatal Exercise Sheets
5. Caesarian Section Exercises
6. Booklist
7. Newsletter—three times per year

Wall Charts—see catalogue book re addresses

1. Birth Books
2. Patient Information Library
3. Childbirth Graphics

Resource centres

Canadian Branch—I.C.E.A.
Linda Ohler
378 Lakeview Avenue
Kingsville, Ontario
N9Y 2E3

Obstetrical Division
Canadian Physiotherapy Association
25 Imperial Street
Toronto, Ontario
M5P 1B9

LaLeche League
LLLI
Canadian Supply Depot
P.O. Box 70
Williamsberg, Ontario
KOC 2H0

Ligue LaLeche du Canada
C.P. 118, Succursale Laval
Ouest Laval, P.Q.
H7R 5B7
— pickup telephone directory for local numbers

Sex Education and Information Council (SIECUS)
Dr M. Barrett
432 Castlefield Avenue
Toronto, Ontario
M5N 1L4

Lamaze Childbirth Association of Ontario
78 Normandy Blvd.
Toronto, Ontario
M4L 3K3

Birthright Montreal
1280 St. Mark Street
Room 204
Montreal, P.Q.
H3H 2G1

Parents of Twins
P.O. Box 3021
Station D
Willowdale, Ontario
M2R 3G5

Books

Note (BB) means books available from Birth Books, P.O. Box 836, Peterbor
Ont.

Cedino, L. (1980) *The Exercise Plus Pregnancy Program: Exercises for Before,
During and After Pregnancy*. New York: William Morrow (BB).

Elkins, V. H. (1980) *The Rights of the Pregnant Parent: How to Have an
Easier, Healthier Hospital Birth together*. Waxwing Productions (BB).

Hotchner, T. (1979) *Pregnancy and Childbirth: A Complete Guide for a New
Life*. New York: Avon Books (BB).

Markowitz, E. (1980) *Baby Dance: A Comprehensive Guide to Prenatal and
Post partum exercise* (BB).

Mendelsohn, R. (1981) *Mal(e) Practice: How Doctors Manipulate Women.*
(BB).

Trimmer, E. *Having a Baby*. Collins

Verny, T. *The Secret Life of the Unborn Child*. Collins (BB).

Reference material

Canadian Institute of Child Health *Prenatal Information in Canada* Resources available on a national basis e.g. pamphlets, books etc on birth
and pregnancy (BB).

Shrock, P. (1980) *Instructional Materials in Childbirth and Parent Education
1-VL* A comprehensive survey of commercial teaching aids, how to make
your own and how to use them effectively. *A Birth and the Family Journal*
reprint (BB).

Stratmeyer *Research in Ultrasound Bioeffects: A Public Health View. New
Birth in the Family Journal* reprint (BB).

SOUTH AFRICA

Compiled by Brenda Kastell

Resource centres

Adoption

Contact any Child Welfare Association:—look under 'C' in your telephone
directory *S.A. National Council for Child Welfare.*
   Tel. (011) 833-7240.

Adoptive Parents Association of S.A.—provides guidance for adoptive parents and children
Tel. (011) 784-3081.

Homes for Unmarried Mothers—some addresses from each province:
Cape
   St Anne's Home Tel. (021) 45-1596
   Nannie Huis Tel. (021) 67-2797

Durban
  Birthright Tel. (031) 31-5306
  St Gabriels Home for Coloureds Tel. (031) 88-2840
Johannesburg
  Princess Alice Adoption Home Tel. (011) 646-5641
  Chris-Magte Tel. (011) 440–5618
  Khulani Girls' Club Soweto

Baby-sitters

Durban
  Rent-a-granny Tel. (031) 85-8086
  Granny services Tel. (031) 86-1577
Johannesburg
  Rent-a-granny Tel. (011) 787-4213
  Serviceable Sisters tel. (011) 788-9302
Some universities have a student baby-sitter service—look under 'U' in the telephone book

Books

All about Childbirth A manual for prepared childbirth by Alice T. Mac-Mahon R. N. Revised S.A. Edition. Published by Waide Heaton
Baby and Child Care Handbook. Complete guide for S.A. parents—including excellent resource section from 'A' to 'W'. This book is a 'first' in S.A. by Marina Petropoulo (Arrangements are in hand for a paperback edition and Afrikaans translation)
Baby's First Year. Published by Waide Heaton. This excellent book is supplied free with a 'Your baby pack' of available samples. Application is made by card supplied by Hospitals, Doctors, Physiotherapists and Nappy packs etc. to Waide Heaton, P.B. 39 102 2018.

Guides to social services

A Guide to Health & Social Services in Johannesburg Area by Avis Schreier. Published by Dept. of Paediatrics Wits. University.
Social Welfare Handbook. A guide to Welfare Agencies of Durban, N. & S. Coast, KwaZu Logan's University Books.
Child Care Information Centre Directory of Services. Rondebosch & Mowbray Children's Centre. 7700

Booklets

For Mothers Who Care by Drs. O. Titze, Germany & K. H. Friedlander, New Zealand,. Published by Natural Health Association of S.A. P.B.39556. 2018
  Natural remedies for pregnancy & babies.
How Does Your Baby Grow 'Hoe Groei U Baba' Published by Lederle

Laboratories—Education Service to Obstetricians & Gynaecologists, for their patients.

You and Your Baby Published by Lay Publications for S.A. Medical Association (Available in English, Afrikaans, Xhosa, Zulu, Sotho, Pedi & Tswana)

These booklets are obtainable free of charge from Hospitals, Doctors & Clinics, or from: Lay Publications, (M.A. of S.A.), Private Bag X1, Pinelands. 7430.

In 1983 *You & Your Baby* will be published in two parts—
Part 1—Conception to Birth: Part II—Birth to two years.

Other Medical Association Publications are listed below:

Be Safe at Home, You and Your Eyes, You and Your Teeth, Coping with Tension, You and Your Doctor, You and Your Marriage, You and Your Skin, Know the Teenager, Home and Personal Hygiene

N.B. Family doctor publications of the British Medical Association are also available.

Booklets and leaflets

Dept. of Health/Dept. van Gesondheid

P.Bag X88, Pretoria.0001   *Diet During Pregnancy & Breast Feeding*
                                  Dieet Tydens Swangerskap en Borsvoeding
Scientific Nutrition and You   Bulletin 4, 5, and 6
Wetenskaplike Voeding en u   Bulletin 4, 5 and 6

Dept. of Health and Welfare/Dept. van Gesondheid en Welsyn

Private Bag X63, Pretoria 0001
Breastfeeding/Borsvoeding
Successful Family Planning/Suksesvolle Geinspb.
Feeding the Young Child/Voeding van die Jong Kind

Dept. of National Education/Dept. van Nasionale Opvoeding

Private Bag X122. Pretoria
Clothing No. 93   *Elegance for the Expectant Mother*
Kleding No. 93   *Lyk Mooi Terwyl U Wag*
Clothing No. 94   *Baby Layette and other Equipment*
Kleding No. 94   *Bab Uitset en ander Toerusting*

Dental Association of S.A./Tandheelkundige van S.A.

Private Bag 1. Houghton 2041
Privaat Sak
Dear Mother To Be/Geagte Aanstaamde Moeder
Your Child's Teeth/U Kind se Tande

Nestle (S.A.) (Pty.) Ltd

P.O. Box 50659. Randburg 2125
Posbus 50659. Randburg 2125
   Antenatal Exercises/Voorgeboorteoefeninge
   Postnatal Exercises/Na Geboorte—Oefeninge
N.B. These exercise sheets are being re-written by the Obstetric Association
of the S.A. Society of Physiotherapy and should be printed early in 1983.

   Catalogue of books on pregnancy and birth and baby and child care can
be obtained by writing to: Birth books, 2 Almondbury Lane, Tokai. 7945.
Tel. (021) 72–1761
   N.B. On joining the Obstetric Association of the S.A.S.P. you will receive a catalogue and have access to *your own library* by post.
Librarian: Mrs Cynthia Bauer, 29 Edward St. Westdene, Benoni. 1500. Tel.
(011) 54–4628
   To add to book list: Lend Baby a Hand by Agnes Wenham MCSP (Johannesburg). Published 1980 by Heinemann, London
   This is an illustrated guide to posture care—Neuman-Neurode's baby
gymnastics and Ortho Toys.

Breast feeding

Breast Feeding Association aims to promote breast feeding by giving support,
advice and encouragement to mothers through free telephone counselling
service, as well as lectures and visits to hospitals.
Cape Peninsula, Tel. (021) 66-8363, answering service provides numbers for
   all suburbs
East London, Tel. (0431) 25887
Stellenbosch, Tel. (02231) 3816
Pretoria. Tel. (012) 46-7337
Port Elizabeth, Tel. (041) 74693
Johannesburg. Tel. (011) 678-3230

La Leche League

National District Advisor—Eve Gray, Northcliff. Johannesburg. Tel. (011)
678–4184
Answering service giving Tel. numbers of six counsellors.
   Johannesburg   Tel. 88-6038—Gail Brown
   Cape Town   Tel. (021) 61-6486
   Belville   Tel. (021) 99-3808
   Port Elizabeth   Tel. (041) 53-1577
   Westville   Tel. (031) 85-9952
   Bloemfontein   Tel. (051) 79446
   Soweto   Tel. (011) 672-9675
   Pretoria   Tel. (012) 83-3926

Childbirth

Antenatal clinics for medical checks, exercises, relaxation and breathing techniques are available at all large hospitals e.g.
Johannesburg Hospital, Tel. (011) 643-0111
Alexandra Health Centre. Tel. (011) 440-1231
Soweto. Tel. (011) 944-3070
Lenasia, Tel. (011) 852-1432
Baragwanath. Tel. (011) 933-3110
Private obstetric physiotherapists. Register obtainable from:
Tel. (012) 44-2070-Secretary of Obstetric Association, 519 Lukas St, Lukasrand. 0181 or Tel. (011) 440-4557-Chairman of Obstetric Association, 26, Desborough Ave, Winston Ridge 2196

Depression

Depression after the birth of a baby is common and anyone who feels that she cannot cope may telephone:

Life line—Cape Town, Durban and Johannesburg
Crisis clinic, Cape Town and Johannesburg
Stress clinic, Johannesburg. Tel. (011) 752-1422

Films on childbirth etc.

This list was prepared by the Obstetric Association of the S.A.S.P. We apologise that all the telephone numbers given below are Johannesburg, code (011). The O.A. would appreciate information on films available in other areas of South Africa.
1. Abbott Laboratories (Makers of Similac) Tel. Mr Welgemoed (Bedford-view Nutrition Br) 53-4520

    3 Films:- *The Amazing Newborn* 25 minutes
    Bonding 25 minutes
    Breastfeeding 25 minutes
2. Glaxo-Allenburys S.A. Tel. Mrs Clements 34-9172—Catalogue available
    Ready for Baby 24 mins.
3. Municipality City Health Dept. Tel. 777–1111—Health Education—Mrs. V. D. Berg
    Library
    2 Films:- *Preparing for Sarah* 20 mins.
    How babies are born 11 mins. Sex education for children—animated.
4. Nestle Tel. Mrs. Appelblom—787–9500
    1 Film:- *First Days of Life* 20 mins.
5. Sandoz Tel. Mrs. Adams—789 1920
    1 Film:- *Normal Delivery* 20 mins.
6. SKF (Smith Kline & French) Tel. Mrs. Steyn—36-7011
    1 Film:- *Birthday*

7. Smith & Nephew
   P.O. Box 92 Pinetown
   3600
   Tel. Airline Peacock—618-2466—for arrangements.
   Film:-   *Birth of a Baby*   35–40 mins.
8. Wyeth Laboratories Tel. Mrs. Rajah 440-4526
   3 Copies—*Birth of a Family*   20–30 mins.

Family planning

Advice on contraception and contraceptives available free or at a nominal cost from all family planning centres. Look under 'F' in the telephone directory.

Parentcraft

This is a new project of the Breast Feeding Association:
Cape Town	Tel. (021) 72-1370
East London	Tel. (0431) 25887
Transvaal-Benoni	Tel. 849-7535 Betty Anne Starkey

Education for birth

Classes for mothers and fathers on all aspects of family centered childbirth—hospital, home and Caesarean.

Patricia Glaumm 2 Almondbury Lane, Tokai. 7945 Tel. (021) 72-1761
Guidance for parents—John and Linda Strydom Tel. (031) 35-2461 Ext. 399. Durban
ICEA—for affiliated groups starting in South Africa contact:
Western Cape. Tel. (021) 96-5200. Eastern Cape. Tel. (0431) 25887
Transvaal and Northern Cape. Tel. (021) 83-2459
Natal. Tel. (031) 93-4122
Swaziland. Pamela Attwell, University College of Swaziland, Private Bag, Kwaluseni, Swaziland.

Slides

No slides have been made on a commercial basis so far in South Africa.

Teaching aids

Birth atlas — Maternity Center Association, 48 East 92nd St, New York
           — Order from Westdene Services (Med. Books) 10028
                Tel. (011) 39-1711
Knitted uterus pattern—copy obtainable from the O.A. for members
Obstetric pelvis — Catalogue No. S.A.M. 52
                         With ligaments

Obtainable from; R. M. Salters, 502 Main Reef Rd. Denver. 2027
P.O. Box 2530. Johannesburg. 2000
Tel. (011) 615-6410
N.B. R. M. Salters used to be Gurr Surgical
Fetal doll with placenta also obtainable from above
Fetal doll (no placenta)
Complete fetal model (pink or brown)
Fetal model kit (pink or brown)
Obtainable from:—Childbirth Graphics, P.O. Box 17025, Irondequoit.
Rochester. N.Y. 14617.

Twins

Mothers of Twins Association of South Africa. Aims to provide emotional
and economic support for mothers of multiple birth children.
Mrs P. Johnson 112, 4th Avenue, Fairlands, Johannesburg 2195. Tel. (011)
678-625

Randburg	Tel. (011) 46-9360
Durban North	Tel. (031) 84-6524
Kimberly	Tel. (0531) 23724
Bloemfontein	Tel. (051) 22-1047
Port Elizabeth	Tel. (041) 30-7284

P.O.T.A.C. Parents Of Twins Association—Mrs Pat Soulsby Tel. (021)
58-13
Gives advice and support to parents of multiple birth children and organises meetings which include fathers.

Index

Abortion, 17
  film about, 248
  prevention of, 88–9
Active birth, 10, 15–16, 167–174
Aids for mothers, 101
Aims of antenatal education, 1, 2–4, 21, 222
  summary of aims, 3–4, 222
Alcohol during pregnancy, 75
Alphafetoprotein measurements, 94–5
Amniocentesis, 93–4
Amnioscopy, 95
Anatomy and physiology, 73–4
Antenatal care
  mother's, 74
  professional, 9, 11, 74
Antenatal examinations, 86–8
Apgar score, 123, 172, 178, 226, 227
Association of Chartered Physiotherapists
  in Obstetrics and Gynaecology, 8, 260
Association of Radical Midwives, 169, 261
Audiovisual aids, 43–56
  address list for, 52–6
  aids from overseas, 285–6
  check list for, 51–2
  choosing, 44–6
  sources of material, 43–4
  useful aids, 46–50
  using, 46

Baby, appearance and activities, 191–5
  films about, 240–6
Baby care, instruction about, 62, 182–190
  bathing, 183
  equipment, 183
  films about, 240–6
  filmstrips about, 255
Baby, newborn, 123, 141, 145, 179
  films about, 240–6

planning for, 184–5
preparing for, 229–30
problems of, 202–3
Backache, 223
Beds
  'borning', 169
  Kings Fund, 169
Bio-feedback machines, 34
Birth, 122–5, 137–45
  'active', 10, 15–16, 167–74
    film about, 249
  films about, 234–40, 249–52, 291
  filmstrips about, 254–5
  history of, 167–9
  of damaged child, 17–18
'Birthing stools', 170
'Bishops score', 152
Bladder, emptying, 86, 132
Blood sampling, fetal, 157
Blood specimens, 89, 91, 95
Blood transfusion, 162
Boards, chalk and other, 46, 185, 212
Books, booklets, leaflets and pamphlets,
  206, 211, 221, 232, 262–4,
  269–70, 276–7, 281–4, 287,
  288–90
Bottle feeding, 184, 185–90
Bowel, emptying, 86
Bradley, Robert A, 16
Breast changes during pregnancy, 183
Breast feeding, 9, 79, 141, 183, 185–90,
  205, 228, 290–1
Breathing, 7, 13, 17, 35, 97, 176–8, 228
  in labour, 122, 127–31, 175
Briance, Prunella, 9

Caesarean section, 15, 90, 158, 160–1
Caldeyro-Barcia, R., 15, 169, 177–8
Catalogues, 284–5
Central Midwives Board, 10, 11
Changes
  emotional, 82

Changes (contd)
  in life style, 3, 82–3, 181, 200–1
  physical, 73–4
Charts, 47, 53–5, 73, 106, 211, 212
Classes, 2, 12, 16–7, 57–70, 223
  accommodation for, 57–9
  addresses for equipment for, 68–70
  antenatal, 105
  couples', 213–4
  equipment for, 57–9
  fathers', 210–3, 231
  outlines for, 64–8
  planning, 59–64
  records and follow-up of, 63–4
  time and duration of, 60–1
Contractions, 15, 110, 113–5, 121–3,
    132–40, 153, 154, 155, 157, 177
  cessation or slowing of, 154–5
Cooperation cards, 86
Counselling, individual, 27–8

Demand feeding, 184
Diagrams, 43, 45, 73, 106, 114
Dickinson-Belskie birth atlas, 53, 73,
    106, 141–145
Dick-Read, Dr Grantly, 6–7, 9, 10, 14,
    15, 111, 225, 263
Diet, 12, 79–82
Domino scheme, 163–4
Drugs
  in labour, 15, 115–21
  in pregnancy, 76

Endorphines, 116
Epidural analgesia, 111, 112, 117–9,
    134, 157–8, 161
Episcopes, 47
Episiotomy, 123, 148–50, 178
Exercises, 19, 21, 31–6, 37, 62, 125–6
  'active' birth, 172–4
  antenatal, 6, 84, 96–100
  postnatal, 6, 198–200, 205

Fairbairn, Dr J.S. and colleagues, 6
Family planning, 12, 18, 203–4, 292
  films about, 246–8
  filmstrips about, 255–6
Family, problems of, 203
Family relationships, 1, 2–3, 180–1,
    197–8
  films about, 240–6
Fathers
  advice to, 218–20
  classes for, 210–3, 231
  evenings, 207–21

information for, 207–13
  role playing, 38
Fear, 7, 33, 71, 111
Fetal development, 12
  models of, 50
Fetal monitoring, 90–1
  film about, 248
  heart monitoring, 90–1, 112, 152,
    155–6
  sonic aid monitoring, 156, 172
Fetal reactions to labour, 155–7
Fetus, position of
  anterior, 157
  breech, 157–8
  posterior, 157
Fibrocystic disease, 193
Film evenings, 214–8
Film loops, 49, 258–9
Films, 43, 44, 47, 48, 76, 109, 198, 200,
    204, 210, 213, 214–7, 234–52,
    271–4, 277–80, 291–2
Filmstrips, 43, 44, 47, 73, 76, 198, 200,
    204, 211, 212, 254–6
Flannelgraphs, 45, 47, 55, 73, 81, 106
Forceps delivery, 158–9

Gas and oxygen inhalation, 117, 122,
    134, 137
Group discussion, 15, 28–31, 34–5, 62,
    76, 81–2, 83–4, 109, 200–2,
    211–3
  'Trigger' films for, 238
Groups in antenatal education, 14, 15,
    28–31, 36, 105
  value of, 229
Guthrie test, 193

Harrison, Sheila, 8, 126, 175, 224
Health visitors, 5–6, 11–12, 19, 44, 88,
    163
Heardman, Helen, 7, 14, 127, 225
History of antenatal education, 4–20
Hormone balance, 89
Hospital bookings, differences in,
    162–5
Husbands, classes for, 16, 231
Hypnosis, 12

Induction, 150–2
Infant feeding, 12, 204
International Childbirth Education
    Association, 15, 267, 286

Jacobsen's 'contrast' method, 32, 97–8
Jaundice, 192–3
Journals, list of American, 265, 281

'Kick chart', 91
Kitzinger, Sheila, 15, 30, 32, 36, 50, 148, 263

Labour, 12, 15, 104–66
  breathing in, 127–31, 175–78
  coping with, 111–13
  effects of antenatal education on, 224–29
  first stage of, 107, 114–5, 121–2
  hospital bookings for, 163
  long, 153
  method of teaching about, 106–8
  middle and late first stage of, 108
  mobility in, 15–16, 17, 156
  normal, 104–46
  onset of, 107
  pain in, 109–11
  physiology of, 108
  precipitate, 154
  pre-labour stage, 107
  premature, 91
  questions about, 106, 110
  rehearsal of, 131–41
  second stage of, 108, 122–4, 167–72
  sensations and reactions in, 109
  short, 153
  third stage of, 108
  variation of patterns in, 147–66
Ladies Health Society, 5
La Leche League, 187, 230, 261, 263, 267, 286, 291
Lamaze, Dr Fernand, and colleagues, 13–14, 128, 226, 263, 286
Layette, 183, 185, 230
Leboyer deliveries, 124–5
  film about, 236
  filmstrip about, 255
Lee Buxton, 14

Madders, Jane, 32
Mandelstam, Dorothy, 8, 222, 223, 225
Maternity care, 165
McEwan, Margaret, 5
Midwives, 10–12, 42, 87, 108, 112, 122, 163–5, 168–9, 222, 224, 260
Mitchell, Laura, 32–4, 127
Models, 44, 49, 50, 52, 73, 107, 114, 212
Mother, problems of, 202
Multigravidae, 3, 60, 84, 109, 163, 180, 200
  classes for, 16–17
Muscle action, 32, 34

National Childbirth Trust, 8, 13, 15, 44, 50, 60, 101, 172, 187, 205, 211, 230, 260
Negative results of antenatal education, 231–2
Neuromuscular control, 31–6, 72–3, 96–100, 125–31
Nitrous oxide analgesia, 120–1

Obstetric Association of Chartered Physiotherapists, 7, 8, 224
Odent, Michel, 15, 111, 169

Pain, 7, 13, 33, 109–11, 114–5, 224, 227, 228
Parentcraft, 292
Parenthood, 1–3, 10, 181, 184
  guidelines for, 18
  Open University course for, 253
  preparation for, 222
  problems of, 181–2, 200–4
Parents' Federation of New Zealand, 15
Pelvis, 49–51, 85–6, 97, 98–9, 211
Pethidine analgesia, 119–20, 134
Phenylketonuria, 193
Phototherapy, 192
Physiotherapists, 6, 7, 8, 44, 59, 88, 198
Pictures, 43, 47, 106
Placenta, 23, 76, 92, 124
  retained, 162
Planning a course, 22–7, 57–69
Playlets in teaching, 39–40
Posters, 47, 82, 259
Postnatal rehabilitation, 14
Postnatal support groups, 9
Posture, 84, 100
Pre-conceptual care, 17–19
Pre-eclampsia, 88, 150
Pregnancy, 71–103
  attitudes to, 1, 2, 71–2
  diet in, 79–81
  dietary problems in, 81
  education about, 1, 12, 72–84
  emotional changes in, 71–2, 82
  fears in, 71
  films about, 234–8
  filmstrips about, 254–5
  health care in, 74–6
  hospital bookings in, 162
  neuromuscular control in, 96–100
  nutrition in, 76–9
  physical changes in, 73–4
  questions about, 72
  sexual relationships in, 83, 86
  timing of teaching about, 100

Pregnancy (contd)
  useful addresses, 103
  weight in, 77, 79
Preinduction, 152
Primigravidae, 3, 60, 84, 109, 164, 180
Problems, behavioural and learning, 293
Projectors, 43, 46
Prostaglandin gel, 152
Psychoprophylaxis, 10, 12–14, 108,
  111, 172, 223, 226–9
  American Society for, 227, 266
Puerperium, 163, 179–82, 184, 195–8
  attitudes to, 179–81
Pushing routine, 121–2, 129–30, 137

Radio-telemetry, 156, 172
Randell, Miss Minnie, 6, 15
Records, 46, 49, 55
Reinforcement, 37
Relaxation, 7, 10, 13, 17, 32–4, 36, 84,
  97–9, 125–7, 262
Respiratory distress syndrome (RDS),
  193
Rhesus factor (Rh), 89, 93, 193
Role-playing, 38–40, 126–7

Schuchardt charts, 73
Shirodkar suture, 88
Slides, 43, 47, 109, 211, 212, 293
  list of, 256–7, 280
  for non-English speaking groups, 258
  with tapes, 257–8
Smoking during pregnancy, 75
Special care nurseries, 193
Spina bifida, 17–18, 94, 95

Stillbirth, 17, 252
Stress incontinence, 224
Surveys on antenatal education, 222–30

Talks, 22–7, 31, 62
Tape recordings, cassettes, 46, 49, 55,
  109, 257–8, 277, 280
Teachers of antenatal education, 4
  films for, 248–54
Teaching aids, 253, 270–1, 293
Teaching techniques, 21–42
  films for teachers, 248–54
  for foreigners, 40–41
  for normal labour, 106–13
Tension, 7, 33, 98, 126–7, 175
Toxaemia, 223
Transcutaneous electro-nerve
  stimulation (TENS), 121
Twins, 92, 95, 162, 293–4

Ultrasonic echo sounding (ultrasound),
  91–3, 150
  film about, 251
Urine testing, 88
Useful addresses, 259–62, 264, 266–9,
  274–5, 287–8
Uterus, 23, 114
  knitted model, 50, 107, 114

Value of antenatal education, 222–233
Vegan mothers, 78
Velvovski, 12, 13
Ventouse vacuum extraction, 159–60
Version, external, 89–90
Video-cassettes about birth, 43, 238–9